THE POLITICS OF POTENTIAL

MEDICAL ANTHROPOLOGY: HEALTH, INEQUALITY, AND SOCIAL JUSTICE

Series editor: Lenore Manderson

Books in the Medical Anthropology series are concerned with social patterns of and social responses to ill health, disease, and suffering and how social exclusion and social justice shape health and healing outcomes. The series is designed to reflect the diversity of contemporary medical anthropological research and writing and will offer scholars a forum for publishing work that showcases the theoretical sophistication, methodological soundness, and ethnographic richness of the field.

Books in the series may include studies on the organization and movement of peoples, technologies, and treatments; how inequalities pattern access to these; and how individuals, communities, and states respond to various assaults on well-being, including from illness, disaster, and violence.

For a list of all the titles in the series, please see the last page of the book.

THE POLITICS OF POTENTIAL

Global Health and Gendered Futures in South Africa

MICHELLE PENTECOST

RUTGERS UNIVERSITY PRESS
New Brunswick, Camden, and Newark, New Jersey
London and Oxford

Rutgers University Press is a department of Rutgers, The State University of New Jersey, one of the leading public research universities in the nation. By publishing worldwide, it furthers the University's mission of dedication to excellence in teaching, scholarship, research, and clinical care.

Library of Congress Cataloging-in-Publication Data

Names: Pentecost, Michelle, 1984– author.
Title: The politics of potential : global health and gendered futures in South Africa / Michelle Pentecost.
Description: New Brunswick : Rutgers University Press, [2024] | Series: Medical anthropology : health, inequality, and social justice | Includes bibliographical references and index.
Identifiers: LCCN 2023018411 | ISBN 9781978837485 (hardback) | ISBN 9781978837478 (paperback) | ISBN 9781978837492 (epub) | ISBN 9781978837508 (pdf)
Subjects: LCSH: Maternal health services—South Africa—Western Cape—Case studies. | Child health services—South Africa—Western Cape—Case studies. | Maternal and infant welfare—South Africa—Western Cape—Case studies. | Medical policy—South Africa—Western Cape—Case studies. | Western Cape (South Africa)—Social conditions—Case studies. | Western Cape (South Africa)—Social policy—Case studies.
Classification: LCC RG966.S38 P46 2024 | DDC 362.19820096873—dc23/eng/20230911
LC record available at https://lccn.loc.gov/2023018411

A British Cataloging-in-Publication record for this book is available from the British Library.

References to internet websites (URLs) were accurate at the time of writing. Neither the author nor Rutgers University Press is responsible for URLs that may have expired or changed since the manuscript was prepared.

♾ The paper used in this publication meets the requirements of the American National Standard for Information Sciences—Permanence of Paper for Printed Library Materials, ANSI Z39.48–1992.

rutgersuniversitypress.org

For Thomas

CONTENTS

FOREWORD

LENORE MANDERSON

The Medical Anthropology: Health, Inequality, and Social Justice series is concerned with the diversity of contemporary medical anthropological research and writing. The beauty of ethnography is its capacity through storytelling to make sense of suffering as a social experience and to set it in context. Central to our focus in this series, therefore, is how social structures, political and economic systems, and ideologies shape the likelihood and impact of infections, injuries, bodily ruptures and disease, chronic conditions and disability, treatment and care, and social repair and death.

Health and illness are social facts: the circumstances of maintaining and losing health are always and everywhere shaped by structural, local, and global relations. Social formations and relations, cultures, economies, and political organizations shape experiences of illness, disability, and disadvantage as much as ecologies do. The authors of the monographs in this series are concerned centrally with health and illness, healing practices, and access to care, but in the different volumes, they highlight the importance of such differences in context as expressed and experienced at individual, household, and wider levels. Health risks and the outcomes of social structures and household economies (for example, health systems factors), as well as national and global politics and economics shape people's lives. In their accounts of health, inequality, and social justice, the authors move across social circumstances, health conditions, geography, and their intersections and interactions to demonstrate how individuals, communities, and states manage assaults on people's health and well-being.

As medical anthropologists have long illustrated, the relationships between social context and health status are complex. In addressing these questions, the authors in this series showcase the theoretical sophistication, methodological rigor, and empirical richness of the field while expanding a map of illness, social interaction, and institutional life to illustrate the effects of material conditions and social meanings in troubling and surprising ways. The books reflect medical anthropology as a constantly changing field of scholarship, drawing on research in such diverse contexts as residential and virtual communities, clinics, laboratories, and emergency care and public health settings; with service providers, individual healers, and households; and with social bodies, human bodies, biologies, and biographies. While medical anthropology once concentrated on systems of healing, particular diseases, and embodied experiences, today the field has expanded to include environmental disasters, war, science, technology, faith, gender-based violence, and forced migration. Curiosity about the body and its vicissitudes remains a pivot of our work, but our concerns are with the location of bodies in social life and with how social structures, temporal imperatives, and shifting exigencies shape life courses. This dynamic field reflects the ethics of the discipline to address these pressing issues of our time.

As the subtitle of the series indicates, the books center on social exclusion and inclusion, social justice, and repair. The volumes in this series illustrate multiple ways that globalization and national and local inequalities shape health experiences and outcomes across space, how economic, political, and social inequalities influence the likelihood of poor health and its outcomes in different settings. At the same time, social and economic relations enable the institutionalization of poverty: they produce the unequal conditions of everyday life and work and hence powerfully influence who gets sick and who is most likely to survive. The books challenge readers to reflect on suffering, deficit, and despair within families and communities while they also encourage readers to remain alert to resistance and restitution—to consider how people respond to injustices and evade the fissures that might seem to predetermine their lives.

In *The Politics of Potential*, Michelle Pentecost examines twenty-first-century understandings of South Africa's increasing prevalence of noncommunicable diseases in the form of obesity and associated metabolic disease. The mounting number of cases of these conditions, which include heart disease and diabetes, has global implications for health and medical services and pharmaceutical costs. In this light, epidemiologists, health economists and health systems specialists found inspiration in the understanding that nutrition prior to conception and during pregnancy influences fetal development and the risk for offspring noncommunicable diseases in adulthood. Both undernutrition and overnutrition in utero predispose an infant to overweight or obesity in adulthood with concomitant metabolic risks that include diabetes, heart disease, and a range of medical complications that follow from these primary conditions. These risks might be transmitted across two generations: grandparents' risk factors might influence their grandchildren's risk of diabetes, heart disease and other conditions.

The policy response has focused on treating both maternal undernutrition in pregnancy for women deemed underweight and preventing excess weight gain via health education for women pregnant who are classified as of normal weight, overweight, or obese according to biometric monitoring. During ordinary antenatal care, such as checking the pregnancy (measuring fundal height, for instance) and testing urine for possible gestational diabetes, women are enjoined to eat well not just for the health of the fetus but for the health of the infant in early childhood and in adulthood, and, in turn, for the health of future generations.

The first antenatal programs were introduced worldwide when the focus was on the proximate risks during pregnancy and childbirth of fetal and maternal death. The antenatal care programs to which women present today have their footings in ideas of maternal and infant care that were introduced in colonial centers in the very early twentieth century. In England, these early interventions were developed in the wake of the loss of young adult men in the Anglo-Boer War and the perception that the country's population was not fit for the needs of industry and defense. A focus on maternal nutrition and education was seen as the route to the health of the nation. These ideas were quickly introduced to colonies (such as South Africa at the time) and to newly independent countries (Davin 1978). More than a century on, women's responsibility for the health of future generations still extends beyond the logic of their pregnancy and their own bodily role in nurturing their growing fetus.

In South Africa and elsewhere, recommendations to breastfeed exclusively have varied in the last few decades as health advisors and researchers worried about the possible risks of HIV infection, but most instructions that women receive when they present for antenatal care are no different from those their mothers and grandmothers received: eat well during pregnancy, breastfeed infants, and ensure good nutrition as they wean and move into childhood. But as Michelle Pentecost illustrates, for the women who are subject to surveillance from conception through pregnancy and in the months afterward—the first 1,000 days—the emphasis has shifted to a powerful focus on the future framed in the language of the developmental origins of health and disease.

Michelle Pentecost begins *The Politics of Potential* with a genealogy of the concept of the first 1,000 days—from conception to about two years after birth—and its centering on mother and child. The first 1,000 days is an idea about how to subvert the growing incidence of cardiometabolic diseases and their comorbidities before the development of disease takes hold. But as Michelle Pentecost takes us from research conferences and stakeholder meetings to clinic to community to home, we see how such an approach is undermined by an exclusive focus on the mother-child dyad and on individual responsibility. The women who are targeted with the personal, embodied responsibility of realizing better health for future generations live in extreme poverty and deprivation and lack access to the money, foods, and other means to realize this goal. Those leading this image of better health overlook the context that diverts potential and thus the impossibility of its realization without major social and structural change.

These policies also overlook the fact that beyond the pregnancy, the mother and her child are not the only people involved in the social reproduction of the infant or in the networks of people around the mother. Infants may be cared for by other people besides their biological mother, perhaps by their mother's mother, their mother's grandmother, an aunt, or the mother of the infant's father. Gender, not the specific relationship, determines who undertakes most of the care work. HIV necessitated this flexibility of configurations of family, in South

Africa and elsewhere. But much earlier, families always had to be flexible because of labor migration, its forced segregation by gender, and further disruptions with labor market entry.

The families in *The Politics of Potential* live with these interpersonal, economic, and social disruptions in a network of townships and informal settlements in Cape Town that are severed from wealthier suburbs by the city's geography. Pentecost's participants hold high aspirations for themselves and their children in relation to health, education, and employment. They long for the privileges that come with relative wealth—a good car, a large enough house, a wide-screen TV, nice clothes. These hopes often crash with unemployment, family rupture, violence, and persistent poverty. In this context, where there is often not enough food for all householders, directives to pregnant women to eat good food and lose weight seem perverse and contrary.

A central problem is, Michelle Pentecost suggests, the problem of responsibility for historical injury. That is, apartheid and its vestiges in contemporary South African society undermine the capacity of women and others in their family to live, eat, and act in ways that would ensure the best possible outcomes for their children. Women struggle to make ends meet in settings where too many people share single-room houses that lack piped water or legal access to power in neighborhoods where the lanes between those houses are always settings of danger. In these areas, good, nutritious, and affordable food of the sort that pregnant women are enjoined to eat is hard to come by. In this skillfully narrated, moving account, Michelle Pentecost peels back the layers that defy individual potential. Colonialism, the vestiges and legacies of apartheid, and administrative incompetence, underfunding, and corruption all undermine quality of care, the capacity to seek it, and the logic of advice.

In *The Politics of Potential*, Michelle Pentecost offers a compelling example of the translation to local settings of shifting knowledge systems in global health. The focus on early life interventions to prevent adult cardiometabolic risk has led to a gendered approach to tackling noncommunicable diseases that pays little attention to the local circumstances of women's lives. The injunctions around maternal weight and fetal and infant nutrition are inevitably gendered because of the obvious biology of reproduction, but structural, situational, and gendered barriers also impact women's capacity to ensure adequate nutrition and health, however defined, within households and across generations.

THE POLITICS OF POTENTIAL

INTRODUCTION

"We were raised by our grandmothers, but now we will have the guts to raise our children." Twenty-four-year-old Nandipha, quite unencumbered by her blooming pregnancy, sat cross-legged in a leather armchair angled toward the sizable television and sound system that dominated her living room. She wore an orange headscarf and a black dress with a fitted bodice embroidered with small red roses. A self-professed fashionista, Nandipha would pair leather dungarees with a red tank top and fluffy pink boots for an ordinary day of housework. For parties, she sported colorfully patterned halter-neck dresses that flare from the waist for swirling around on the dance floor. Even casually dressed, she exuded her own hyper-urban style—Puma trainers, black sweatpants, an oversized sweater, and a bright headscarf. Her mother was a dressmaker. "It was her desire that I be a fashion designer," Nandipha said.

Born in 1990, Nandipha was raised by her grandparents in the Eastern Cape province of South Africa while her mother worked in Cape Town's garment manufacturing industry, a sizeable employer of young women in the city at that time. After completing her secondary education in the Eastern Cape, Nandipha moved to Cape Town to live with her mother, who had married for a second time and had two more children. Nandipha's relationship with her mother and her second family, as Nandipha called them, was fraught. Nandipha had seen little of her mother while growing up in her grandparents' home and did not feel welcome in her mother's new family. Shortly after the move to Cape Town, she left to stay with her uncle. Soon afterward, she met her partner Busi and moved in with him. A short while later she was pregnant with their first child. I met her in 2014 at her first antenatal visit at her local clinic in Khayelitsha.

Nandipha and Busi lived in an established suburb of Khayelitsha, Cape Town's largest township.[1] Unlike many Khayelitsha residents, who live in informal housing without amenities, Nandipha and Busi rented a brick house with an indoor toilet and running water. Busi worked for a travel agent and commuted forty-five minutes one way by minibus taxi to Cape Town's central business district every day, while Nandipha did the housework. She wanted to study graphic design and planned to enroll at a local college the following year to obtain a qualification.

Busi was very supportive of this goal. "This year, we are planning for her to go back to school," he said. "I don't want her to sit at home and do nothing. She also has her dreams that she needs to follow. Housewives are not in fashion!"

Busi was a people person: garrulous, jovial, and warm. He doted on Nandipha and had a clear vision for their future together. They would get married and have another child in six or seven years once they had "sorted her career." He was ecstatic about the pregnancy. He had one daughter from a previous marriage and was hoping for a boy. "Every child is a blessing, although I am praying for a boy. . . . Every man is praying for a boy! Us African men, we need a boy in our lives! Although every child is my blood, in truth I am praying for a boy, and she is praying for a girl!"

It was Busi who worried about getting Nandipha a South African identity document (ID) so she could register to study and access the state child support grant once the baby was born. Nandipha's birth certificate and ID had been misplaced by the time she finished high school, and she had attempted to apply for both in the Eastern Cape. She had received the birth certificate, but it had mistakes related to her name and date of birth. She had applied for a new birth certificate and ID but had moved to Cape Town before the latter arrived. In Cape Town, officials noted that she had applied in the Eastern Cape and would not process a new application. It had been six years since she had made the application in the Eastern Cape. Busi had spent countless hours telephoning the Department of Home Affairs to resolve the problem. He hoped that if he "phoned and bothered" them enough, they would sort it out. He continued to phone them throughout Nandipha's pregnancy to no avail. It took the help of a colleague who had previously worked at Home Affairs to finally secure Nandipha's credit-card-sized proof of identity some months after the birth of their child. Nandipha described it as "like winning a prize" because it permitted her to apply for college, apply for a child support grant, get a bank account, obtain her driver's license, and vote in elections.

During her pregnancy, Nandipha cleaned the house, watched television, listened to music, and read her small collection of magazines and books. Her taste was eclectic. Titles on the bookshelf ranged from inspirational religious texts to *Bitch Please! I'm Khanyi Mbau* (Mofokeng 2012), a tell-all autobiography of South Africa's self-proclaimed Queen of Bling. Like most of its critics, Nandipha panned it. By contrast, she had high praise for the dog-eared copy of *Disgrace* (Coetzee 1999) on her coffee table. I noticed it and asked her what she had made of it. "This was a good one," she said, picking it up slowly and tracing her finger on the cover. "That lecturer was sleeping with his students," she said, shaking her head. She replaced it on the shelf and changed the subject when I asked her what she thought about the book's ending.

Published in 1999, Coetzee's *Disgrace* is set in the early post-apartheid era and tells the fictional story of David Lurie, an aging White professor who is dismissed from his post at a Cape Town university after pursuing a sexual relationship with Melanie Isaacs, one of his female students, who brings a formal complaint. Although Melanie's race is ambiguous in the text, during the university hearings, it is implied that Lurie's transgressions continue racialized and gendered patterns of exploitation. Coetzee uses the hearings to invoke questions of the limits of law and the possibilities of reconciliation against the implicit backdrop of the hearings of the national Truth and Reconciliation Commission (TRC), which had sought to gather information about human rights violations during apartheid and facilitate amnesty, reparations, and reconciliation. In the book, Lurie admits guilt but refuses to apologize. He rejects the hearing committee's conclusion that he has failed to see his actions within the context of a "long history of exploitation" (Coetzee 1999, 53). In a state of disgrace, Lurie retreats to his daughter's farm in the Eastern Cape, where the rural peace is soon shattered by an attack on the property and the gang rape of Lurie's daughter Lucy. Lucy becomes pregnant and resolves to stay on the farm, to Lurie's consternation. He suspects that Petrus, the Black owner of a neighboring farm, was behind the attack, and that in staying Lucy is tacitly offering her land in exchange for Petrus's protection.

Coetzee's juxtaposition of these two events of sexual violence is often read as a rebuke of Lurie's refusal of responsibility, but literary scholar Stefanie Boese argues that such a reading overlooks the very different historical and social coordinates of these events. Boese (2017, 248) is concerned with "temporality as a crucial, if easily overlooked, dimension of social justice struggles." Lurie's hearing committee, Boese points out, has no legal avenue that might frame his actions in the longue durée[2] of White colonial violence. Similarly, the TRC's focus on spectacular acts of violence was inadequate to account for the longstanding systemic injuries of colonial and apartheid rule. Temporality, as Boese argues, is an essential lens for viewing "the embodied afterlives of the colonial encounter" (255).

I had read *Disgrace* more than ten times as an assigned text during my expensive private school education in the heart of the Cape Winelands, in a classroom about fifteen kilometers from Nandipha's home. My upbringing was that of a privileged White South African. I was 10 years old at the inauguration of the democratic era and I only began to fully understand the vastly unequal life outcomes for Black and White South Africans during the medical training and clinical work I pursued after high school.[3] While my medical education was pointedly ahistorical—an education in narrowing the gaze, sidelining the social and the political in order to foreground what could be deemed biomedical (Pentecost 2018a)—the patterning and distribution of illness I encountered was clear. The disease burden was disproportionately borne by poor people, and that group was disproportionately Black as the result of centuries of racism—from slavery and colonialism to apartheid and the perpetuated racial inequities of the post-apartheid era.

Coetzee's focus on "the problem of responsibility toward historical injury" (Boese 2017, 252) is, in many ways, also the problem that animates this book. The better and worse ways in which responsibility toward historical injury is recognized in South Africa is reflected in state policy, in the provision of health care, and in collective and individual visions of citizenship.

This book is about the question of intergenerational responsibility for health and prosperity. As the stories told here will show, this is increasingly understood as an individual mandate in response to new scientific ideas about intergenerational transmissions of the risk of health and disease and human capital—a shift that elides acknowledgment of the systemic factors that structure intergenerational patterns of inequalities in health and well-being.

Nandipha was one of fifteen women I came to know in 2014–2015. I met them in Khayelitsha during their antenatal care visits at their local clinics as part of ethnographic fieldwork that focused on how a new global initiative to focus on nutrition during the first 1,000 days of pregnancy and infancy was implemented in South Africa. The focus on nutritional interventions during the first 1,000 days of life—the period between conception and a child's second birthday—reflects evolving scientific understanding of the impact of early life exposures on health and disease outcomes in adulthood. Since 2013, South Africa's nutrition policy, in partnership with the World Health Organization, UNICEF, and the Global Alliance in Nutrition, has endorsed a "lifecycle approach, focusing on the key 'window of opportunity,' namely pregnancy and the first two years of life (the first 1000 days)" (Department of Health 2013a, 16).

A catchy and convenient shorthand, the concept of the first 1,000 days has shaped nutrition and early life policy in over forty countries. The target of first 1,000 days policies is malnutrition in pregnancy and early childhood, including both undernutrition and overnutrition, based on the notion that poor nutrition has long-term risks for obesity and noncommunicable diseases in adulthood. In the logic of first 1,000 days interventions, breastfeeding promotion, health education during pregnancy, and nutrition supplementation during pregnancy and in early childhood would be the keys to ensuring health and also the means by which economic prosperity and the future could be secured. The elegant simplicity of the concept—just get it right in the first 1,000 days and a healthy, prosperous future awaits—has ensured its international popularity and uptake in government programs, nongovernmental initiatives, and global philanthropies.

In this book, I trace how the first 1,000 days concept shaped policy in the Western Cape province of South Africa from 2013 to 2015, examining its material effects on post-apartheid state policies, clinical care, and the lives of childbearing women in South Africa. To understand the implementation and implications of first 1,000 days policies, I spent fifteen months engaging with South African scientists, policymakers, and clinicians as well as with Nandipha and fourteen other women. My fieldwork spanned these women's pregnancies and the first six months of their infants' lives.

As Nandipha's exclamation that she will "have the guts" to raise her children illustrates, the first 1,000 days message resonates in complex ways in a country where capacity to tend to intergenerational ties and obligations has long been shaped by histories of displacement, disenfranchisement, and staggering inequality. Through an ethnographic analysis of the first 1,000 days initiative in South Africa, I examine how such complexities of intergenerational responsibility are parsed and passed over in policy and practice. Certain framings of perceived global health concerns have had public and political salience, while others have not. Why was the first 1,000 days project so readily adopted by South Africa and many other countries? What do the values and discourses that underpin the first 1,000 days intervention and its instantiation in South Africa and elsewhere reveal about the field of global health in the early twenty-first century? How has the clinical practice of perinatal care in South Africa in the 2010s, as in many other contexts, been shaped by the measurement, categorization, audit, and evaluation that have characterized the global health era? What are the implications of those practices for how responsibility is construed individually rather than collectively? How does the futurity of the first 1,000 days vision accord with the local realities of the women and children who are the targets of such policies?

I trace the first 1,000 days project in South Africa to tell a story that illustrates the particular assemblages—semiotic, material, and social—that have constituted the role of South African science in global health in the twenty-first century. The first 1,000 days project is emblematic of the global health era, and Khayelitsha is a site of particular significance for global health projects on the African continent. I examine the disjunctures between the perinatal directives of maternal and child health policies, people's gendered projections of the future for themselves and their children, and the immediacies that structure the everyday, to reveal the powerful notions of potential that circulate in and constitute social life.

BODIES, ECONOMIES, FUTURES

"Malnutrition corrodes the body, the economy and the future." This slogan from 1000days.org, one of many nongovernmental organizations (NGOs) that promotes public health interventions in the first 1,000 days of life, summarizes the logic of the intervention—that optimizing nutrition in early life would not only prevent childhood malnutrition but would also shape long-term risks for noncommunicable diseases in adulthood and produce future human capital.

As a palatable and easy-to-promote slogan that encapsulates the contemporary scientific consensus on nutrition, the first 1,000 days approach has been widely endorsed internationally. The World Health Organization supports it, as do the UN's Scaling Up Nutrition program, UN member countries, and eighty nongovernmental, donor, and private sector partners, the largest of which is the Bill & Melinda Gates Foundation. The significant international energy focused on the first 1,000 days thus exemplifies early twenty-first-century global health projects: it is a transnational enterprise orchestrated by a diverse set of public and private partnerships that are characterized by an imperative to act for the sake of population health, economic development, and humanitarian concern.

Yet the first 1,000 days initiative is not simply another iteration of the maternal-child health interventions that have been a focus of the international and global health eras. Notably, investment in the first 1,000 days is underpinned by revised notions of heredity and intergenerational risk that constitute a new biomedical regime. A focus on early life interventions is one expression of a shift in epidemiological approaches to noncommunicable disease that incorporate new scientific knowledge in the fields of epigenetics and the developmental origins of health and disease (DOHaD).

DOHaD scientists are interested in the "non-genomic transgenerational inheritance of disease risk," or the risk of noncommunicable diseases due to environmental factors during early development (Gluckman et al. 2007, 145). The proposed mechanism of this risk is epigenetic, which is commonly defined in molecular biology as the mechanism by which environmental inputs modulate genetic material and gene expression without changes to DNA (Godfrey et al. 2007). One of the most well-known scientists of epigenetics, Moshe Szyf, summarizes these ideas as follows:

> The idea that inherited genotypes define phenotypes has been paramount in modern biology. The question remains, however, whether stable phenotypes could be also inherited from parents independently of the genetic sequence per se. Recent data suggest that parental experiences can be transmitted behaviorally, through in utero exposure of the developing fetus to the maternal environment, or through either the male or female germline. The challenge is to delineate a plausible mechanism. In the past decade it has been proposed that epigenetic mechanisms are involved in multigenerational transmission of phenotypes and transgenerational inheritance. The prospect that ancestral experiences are written in our epigenome has immense implications for our understanding of human behavior, health, and disease. (Szyf 2015, 134)

For DOHaD scientists interested in understanding the origins of noncommunicable diseases, the implications include turning the lens on the possible effects of nutrition in early life, and South African scientists working in DOHaD have played an influential role in formalizing this field (Norris and Richter 2016).

DOHaD hypotheses have directly informed a global health focus on nutrition during pregnancy and the first two years after birth (Victora et al. 2008), and while there is substantial epidemiological research on interventions in the first 1,000 days, there has been little interrogation of what the significance of these interventions in the early life period might mean for the people who are the target of such a policy focus. Much has been written about how epigenetic and DOHaD science has recast the pregnant body as an "epigenetic vector" (Richardson 2015) that places individual responsibility on pregnant women for preventing future obesity (Warin 2012) and reinscribes racialized and gendered inequalities (Valdez and Deomampo 2019; Valdez 2021). In this book, I am concerned with how such ideas land in the regions of the world where there is the perceived need for such interventions, what I have termed DOHaD geographies (Pentecost 2018b). These regions are often glossed as the Global South, a shorthand that has come to be a hallmark of the language of global health (Khan et al. 2022). Alongside important work in Guatemala (Yates-Doerr 2011), Mexico (Saldaña-Tejeda and Wade 2019), India (Nichols 2019), and Indigenous Australia (Warin et al. 2022), I examine the specific affective and political articulations of postgenomic temporalities in the South African postcolony.

A POLITICS OF POTENTIAL

The DOHaD and epigenetic understandings of disease causation that underpin the first 1,000 days concept depart from prevailing models in three important ways. First, in these frameworks there is no clear-cut dichotomy between conditions that have a genetic basis (congenital) and conditions that are caused by environmental factors (acquired) (Lock and Palsson 2016). The binary gene/environment framework that characterized approaches to disease etiology in the late twentieth century no longer holds, and there is variation in how scientists and epidemiologists conceptualize the environment. In many cases the mother-infant dyad, or the consumption of food, becomes a proxy for "environment" so that experiments or interventions can be effectively designed and executed.[4] Second, DOHaD and epigenetic logic stretches the temporal epidemiological relationship between exposure and outcome to include multiple generations that might be implicated in the transgenerational transmission of disease. Third, these new configurations of exposure and outcome alter the ways scientists and policymakers conceive of and articulate risk.

While risk has been a key framework of modernity (Douglas 1992; Beck 1992) and persists as a central logic of the governance of life in the twenty-first century (Rose 2007), the first 1,000 days approach exemplifies an alternative logic of potential. Potentiality can be defined as a capacity for plasticity, as a latent force that will manifest in a predetermined manner, or as an energy whose direction is open to manipulation and choice (Taussig et al. 2013). It differs from risk in its ambiguity and its inclusion of speculation, expectation, and promise. While the notion of risk that orients global health biosecurity attempts to anticipate the "gap that cannot be known," (Caduff 2014, 302), the concept of potential that DOHaD and epigenetic imaginaries invoke "indexes a gap between what is and what might, could or even should be" (Taussig et al. 2013, 10). This authorises forms of evidence otherwise anathema to the evidence hierarchy of the global health era. The rationale for intervention is not based on randomised-controlled-trial gold standard evidence, but on large correlational studies much lower down on the traditional evidence tree. Paradoxically then, risk calculation in the epigenetic era relies less on evidence-based medicine, and more on a kind of "probabilistic information"—a "divination of the future" (Lock 2005: 52). The first 1,000 days project exemplifies this future-focused global health agenda.

My central argument in this book is that the first 1,000 days initiative illustrates what I term a *politics of potential*. A politics of potential characterizes new investments in global health interventions for maternal and child health and noncommunicable diseases, targeting specific groups and particular geographies with a distinctly future-oriented framework.

The politics of potential has three premises. The first is that *the substance of potential lies in particular places and not in others*. The first 1,000 days concept centers on the mother-child dyad in the context of "transitioning societies' as the key target of DOHaD interventions while excluding a range of other social actors. Through ethnographic encounters at international conferences and in lecture theaters, government offices, clinics, and the homes of my participants, I illustrate how the first 1,000 days concept moves across these spaces and how its assumptions permit its inscription and translation.

The second premise is that *the manifesting of potential is presumed to be an individual responsibility rather than of collective or structural forces*. This premise assumes that the capacity to realize potential can be biometrically categorized, measured, and protected through interventions. As the clinic ethnography will show, through its focus on pregnant women and early childhood, early life nutrition policy in South Africa reflects a global health imperative to enumerate and classify in order to intervene while reinforcing a notion of individual responsibility for a host of health outcomes for present and future generations.

Finally, *potential is framed from the perspective of an already given future end and not from the perspective of the durative present*.[5] The first 1,000 days concept assumes that action in the present is configured by the distant actualization of potential and not by overlooked potentialities that are always already existing and persistent. Through ethnographic attention to how the future encapsulated in the first 1,000 days project articulates with other potentialities that shape my interlocutors' social landscapes, I show how the common set of aspirations around health, education, and the achievement of middle-class status that my participants expressed for themselves and their children were held in tandem with fears related to the possibility of violence and the potential for a child's future to be disrupted by hunger, abuse, drug addiction, induction into a gang, or incarceration. Accounts of violence and how it structures action and life in Khayelitsha point to anticipation in a different register, shaping kinship and intergenerational relations in distinctly gendered ways.

Returning to the core problem—*the problem of responsibility toward historical injury*—a politics of potential situates the question of responsibility in specific individuals in specific places. By focusing on the future, a politics of potential excludes the social and historical coordinates—including colonialism, apartheid legacy, and persistent racialized inequality—that structure the present.

ETHNOGRAPHY IN THE CLINIC AND ELSEWHERE

My interest in the first 1,000 days as a global health strategy for combatting adult noncommunicable diseases had its origins in my clinical work. In 2003–2008, I studied medicine at the University of Cape Town. My training coincided with the protracted fight between the administration of Thabo Mbeki, who denied that HIV caused AIDS, and activist groups, including the Treatment Action Campaign and Médecins Sans Frontières, that worked toward the state provision of antiretroviral medication, which eventually began in 2006.[6] I was well prepared to practice medicine in the era of HIV, but as I worked in Cape Town's public sector from 2009, I witnessed the brutal effects of the confluence of HIV and noncommunicable diseases and learned first hand about the difficulties of managing them as comorbidities.

In the twenty-first century, noncommunicable diseases, including obesity, hypertension, diabetes, and cardiovascular disease, have increased significantly in South Africa (Steyn et al. 2006). In 2018, the World Health Organization estimated obesity rates of 15 percent in the male population and 40 percent in the female population of South Africa (World Health Organisation 2018), and it is predicted that in 2030 nearly 33 percent of the country's children will be classified as obese—the largest anticipated increase in childhood obesity by 2030 of all countries globally (World Obesity Federation 2019). The impacts on the burden of disease for South Africa are already clear. Excess body weight is a contributing factor to 38 percent of cardiovascular disease, 45 percent of ischemic strokes, 68 percent of hypertensive cases, and 87 percent of type 2 diabetes mellitus cases (Joubert et al. 2007).

The provision of antiretrovirals was in many ways the magic bullet it was anticipated to be: they are a simple, effective way to keep people with HIV alive. Yet scholars who have traced the evolution of the HIV epidemic make plain the complexities that have accompanied that breakthrough.[7] As medical students we were taught that noncommunicable diseases were related to "lifestyle" risk factors in adulthood, and we learned about interventions to produce behavior changes related to nutrition and physical activity—interventions of questionable effectiveness. The first 1,000 days presents another magic bullet of sorts.

Targeting nutrition interventions during this critical window of early life seems to be a simple and cost-effective way to achieve a host of outcomes: decrease child undernutrition, prevent adult noncommunicable diseases, and increase future human capital. The simplicity and beauty of the concept is appealing as an intervention against a host of future ills and as a positive action for the creation of a better future. Yet there are unintended effects of a focus on early life for preventing noncommunicable diseases, and significant differences between the global health vision of the first 1,000 days and its actual implementation.

This book is based on an ethnographic study conducted in policy, clinic, and community sites in the Western Cape province of South Africa. Fieldwork took place from September 2013 to November 2015, including fifteen consecutive months from July 2014 to September 2015. My years of work experience as a medical doctor in Khayelitsha and the wider Cape metropole facilitated access to policymakers, health care facility managers, and antenatal clinics and their staff. Interactions with policymakers, health care officials, academics, and NGO employees were crucial for understanding the formulation and implementation of the new nutrition policy. Scientific conferences, workshops, and presentations by academics and policy officials provided opportunities to study the rhetoric and agendas of different actors in the chain between concept, policy, and implementation and to understand the place of South Africa and Cape Town in particular in the production of "African global health."

The bulk of my time was spent in Khayelitsha, a township the apartheid state established in 1983 in an effort to consolidate the African population of Cape Town 30 kilometers away from the city. The plan for Khayelitsha reflected the spatial logic of apartheid, which sought to segregate race groups for "separate development" (Dewar and Watson 1984). As discussed in chapter 3, those geographies of exclusion persist today in the high rates of unemployment in Khayelitsha and the sidelining of many of the township's residents from the formal socioeconomic activities of the city. Khayelitsha's significant burden of disease has made it a key site in Cape Town's "research archipelago" (Rottenburg 2009; Geissler 2013b), where many research projects are orchestrated by a mix of state, NGO, academic, and philanthropic actors. I spent four months in Khayelitsha's antenatal clinics with the help of my research assistant Nomsa.[8] I met with fifteen women and their families in their homes weekly or fortnightly throughout their pregnancies and for the first few months of their infants' lives.

The clinic—both a physical place and an idea or a practice enacted across multiple sites—is a key interface between nutrition policy and its intended targets.[9] The provision of antenatal care in the Western Cape province is based on a decentralized district-based model of primary, secondary, and tertiary levels of care, Most services are provided at primary or district level. The Western Cape has five rural and four urban districts. Khayelitsha is a subdistrict of the Khayelitsha and Eastern District. Antenatal services in Khayelitsha are provided by two midwife and obstetric units and three basic antenatal care clinics. Free services are provided to residents in each facility's catchment area and most residents have a clinic within a few kilometers of their homes. Whether a higher-risk pregnancy is referred to the district, secondary, or tertiary level depends on the requirement for specialized care. Cape Town City Health granted permission for me to conduct research in two clinics—Sunrise Clinic and Kunye Clinic—that offer antenatal services in Khayelitsha.[10] From August to December 2014, I conducted participant observation in these clinics, and interviewed fifteen staff members (doctors and nurses).

The limitations of interviews for understanding health systems and the problems of interviewing health professionals are well documented (Lambert and McKevitt 2002). As Frédéric Le Marcis and Julien Girard note in their ethnography of a South African hospital, health professionals present their "care ideology" when discussing their work—the "values, duties, tasks and responsibilities" that define their roles, but that ideology might be quite disconnected from their actual daily work (Le Marcis and Girard 2015, 163). Having practiced as a medical doctor for several years, I had intimate knowledge of the compartmentalized nature of medical work and of how practitioners are trained to filter out social context (Pentecost 2018a). I knew that much more might be gleaned from triangulating interviews with informal discussions and participant observation of what happened or did not happen—what Le Marcis and Girard refer to as "enacted ethics" (2015, 164). My participant observation included sitting in the waiting room, which was a useful space for having conversations with patients, clinic staff, visiting researchers, teachers, and students and for observing the flow of people, medications, folders, and food through the clinics. I frequently had conversations with staff in the corridors and during lunch hours in the staff room. I sat in on morning staff meetings, attended health promotion sessions, and joined the weekly breastfeeding support groups. I elected not to study the clinical encounter or clinical records to avoid being cast in a clinical role.

I met the women who were the recipients of early life interventions at these clinics. I invited them to take part in a study that would span their pregnancies and the months after birth. My assistant Nomsa and I spent most of our time with fifteen women: Nandipha, Bathandwa, Lumka, Nobomi, Fezeka, Anele, Lindiwe, Inam, Songezwa, Ndileka, Aviwe, Khanyiswa, Nocawe, Veliswa, and Nonyameko.[11] Our first meeting included taking a life history. After that, we rotated between the participants for weekly or fortnightly meetings. Some participants worked part time, and our meetings with them were arranged accordingly. Those who didn't work spent most of their time at home. Nomsa and I would customarily arrive sometime after 10 A.M. and spend around three hours engaging in whatever activities were taking place that day. These would include activities such as cleaning, doing laundry, cooking, shopping, taking care of children, engaging in entrepreneurial work, watching television, attending the clinic, studying, and completing schoolwork. Often the day would be marked by a visit from participants' family members, friends, partners, or neighbors. I saw participants reach the end of their pregnancies and deliver infants that we had the pleasure of meeting in the first few weeks of their lives. By the end of fieldwork, those infants were eight to eleven months old. Over the course of a year, I was able to form a picture of a household's everyday routine, with the caveat that the birth of a child profoundly interrupted those routines and established new ones.

In our discussions, the word "community" was used to describe the local neighborhood and neighbors. Anthropologists have long critiqued concepts of community and the relative weakness of this term as an analytical tool (Guyer 1981; Thornton and Ramphele 1989), yet "community" remains a key term in the global health vocabulary (McKay 2018a) and was used frequently by my interlocutors. I therefore use the term loosely to describe everyday life outside the clinic.[12]

I chose Khayelitsha to study the first 1,000 days initiative for several reasons. From a biomedical perspective, Khayelitsha's health profile is typical of the pattern of intergenerational metabolic disease that the first 1,000 days policy focus seeks to alleviate: child undernutrition coexists with adult obesity and associated noncommunicable diseases, even within the same households (Bourne et al. 1994; Mvo et al. 1999). I also wanted to understand how and in what ways the diverse set of global health actors at work in Khayelitsha might embed the first 1,000 days concept in practice. This vantage point offers a picture of global health that does not conform to what Nolwazi Mkhwanazi (2016) has identified as the "single story" of health and medicine in Africa. As Mkhwanazi argues, the "single story" frequently features an inadequate state health system and a distrust between the African country and its former colonizers, between the people and the state, or among the people themselves. It also is often characterized by the narrative that in the end Africans will overcome these issues by finding "African solutions to African problems" (197, quoting Oxlund 2014, 77). In contrast to this dominant picture of "African global health" in medical anthropology—of innovative top-down global health initiatives in the shadow of failed or receded states— the ecology of global health as viewed from Khayelitsha reveals a far more complex set of stories about medicine, the state, and coloniality in Africa today.

THE PROBLEM OF RESPONSIBILITY TOWARD HISTORICAL INJURY

One's reasons for what one does and what one studies are complex and mostly not articulable even to oneself. It is important to say that I did not write this book out of a desire to privilege a particular perspective or to repeat a particular story. Nevertheless, the writer/ethnographer is also a character in the story. As J. M. Coetzee notes,

To write is to awaken countervoices within oneself, and to dare enter into dialogue with them. As consciousnesses trapped in bodies, communicating with the imperfect tool of language, we often use stories to convey information—to reach toward some sort of truth—and yet because we have no objective access to other consciousnesses, what we are left communicating are stories about ourselves. We are all one self full of countervoices telling stories and seeking truths. (quoted in Attwell 1992, 65)

Coetzee's foregrounding of the ethical has opened fertile paths for ethnographers seeking to understand the problem of care and responsibility in contexts of injustice.[13] Veena Das (2016, 168) asks: "If the present conditions of our life are framed by practices of violence perpetrated through the apparatus of the state with the connivance of citizens, then what kind of responsibility devolves on us, as members of such political communities, even if we have not given our explicit consent to such projects of spectacular or hidden violence?" Any interrogation of intergenerational responsibility is always also a "story about ourselves" and, as Das terms it, is about "the boundaries of the 'We'" (168). In the South African context, Melissa Steyn's (2001, xxxv) articulation is most succinct: "As a White South African I am greatly implicated in racism and structural privilege; I am part of what I study."

I acknowledge my whiteness in this story: a "location of structural advantage," not a "transhistorical essence" but "a complexly constructed product of local, regional, national and global relations, past and present" (Frankenberg 1993, 237). White skin remains a forceful invocation of power relations and colonial histories (Fox 2012) in the field, in the academy (Nyamnjoh 2012), and in the clinic. As physician-anthropologist Clare Wendland describes in her ethnography of medical training in Malawi, "doctors' bodies are perceived as White, and medicine is conceived of as a construction of global whiteness that surpasses national identity" (Wendland 2010, 13, see also Anderson 2003). In Khayelitsha's clinics, biomedicine's covert conflation of "the normal" with "unmarked whiteness" (Anderson 2003) was most evident in posters and promotional material that depicted White health care professionals attending to Black African patients (Figure 1). In the clinic, I was always identified as a doctor. The challenge for this project was thus the continuous negotiation of a deep contradiction: the acknowledgment that whiteness is deeply implicated in the local/global power relations of the postcolony and the simultaneous appropriation of this power for the co-construction of new subjectivities of whiteness through engagement.

To be both physician and participant-observer is not novel. Dual training in medicine and anthropology is increasingly common (Wendland 2019), but an examination of physician-anthropologists reveals two very different positions in work on "global health." Bridget Hanna and Arthur Kleinman (2013, 16) define the "physician-anthropologist" as offering a distinct perspective that uses medical

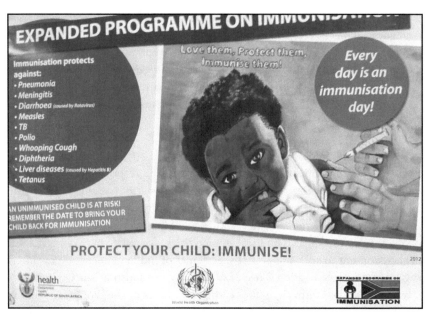

FIGURE 1. Clinic poster. (Photographed by the author, August 2014. © 2014 National Department of Health, Republic of South Africa)

anthropological methods "to hone a vision of health equity and social justice." They offer the examples of Paul Farmer and Jim Yong Kim, physician-anthropologists who cofounded the NGO Partners in Health. By contrast, Didier Fassin points out the ease with which anthropologists with a medical background might adopt global health rhetoric and the moral stance it conveys. He challenges medical anthropologists to "recognize the fine line between scientific detachment and moral involvement" in critical global health research (Fassin 2012a, 114).

These different views reflect a long conversation in anthropology about the place of advocacy and activism in the discipline, under the rubrics of "applied," "public," and "engaged" anthropology (e.g., Hastrup et al. 1990; Singer 1995; Susser 2010; Baer 2012; Hopper 2013), which has particular inflections in South Africa (Gillespie and Dubbeld 2007; Morreira 2012; Nyamnjoh 2015). While I hold Kleinman's (1995) view of the margin between medicine and anthropology as a productive and vital space, I take seriously Fassin's contention that "our sole legitimacy to speak and our sole claim to be listened to depend on our capacity to contest the untested assumptions, the most insidious being that on which we found our moral certainties" (Fassin 2012a, 115). Consequently, I align more closely with Michael Osterweil's perspective on engagement, not as "something we do 'out there'" but rather as a form of critical self-reflection that recognizes and questions the common ideologies and epistemologies in which our practice is situated (2013, 617). For medicine in South Africa, this needs to include a deep reckoning with the historical legacies that still shape medical practice in South Africa today and that all too frequently prevent the possibility of healing.

Like biomedicine, anthropology has a complex history in South Africa and is portrayed as a discipline in crisis, one that is still reckoning with its uncomfortable historical alignments with colonialism and the apartheid project (Gillespie and Dubbeld 2007) and with how it might contribute to social transformation (Susser 2010). Following her time in the townships of Cape Town in 1993–1994, Nancy Scheper-Hughes invoked the theological image of ethnographer as "witness" in her call for anthropology to be "ethically grounded" such that it might act as a "tool for human liberation in the new South Africa" (Scheper-Hughes 1995, 410). But problems arise in casting the ethnographer in the role of "central moral character" (Ong 1995, 430). As Gillespie and Dubbeld (2007) point out, such a position is itself historically situated, and anthropology in South Africa is better served by critical engagement that finds the lines between criticism and activism, or theory and action, necessarily blurred because critical scholarship is itself a political act.

Neither the medic nor the anthropologist is free of the problem of responsibility toward historical injury. The problem will not be resolved in these pages. Rather, naming it as such is an attempt to avoid a "liberal humanism and its anthropological register of ethnographic sentimentalism" (Jobson 2020, 259) in favor of a radical humanist approach that fully acknowledges the coordinates of settler colonialism, apartheid, and global power relations in which this project is situated.

Foregrounding these coordinates is also necessary when faced with the task of writing about violence. Despite my clinical experiences of dealing with high volumes of trauma in South Africa, I was unprepared for the "everydayness of violence" (Nordstrom and Robben 1995, 3) that my interlocutors shared and communicated. As a clinician, I had dealt with the aftermath of violence in Khayelitsha many times in the relatively sanitized confines of the casualty unit. In the field, I discovered that violence and its effects could not be neatly boxed into a diagnosis and a treatment plan. There is no warning, no framework. It is, in Allen Feldman's words, an "ethnographic emergency," where "mental maps go a-kilter, where all things are askew. . . . The ethnographer, like any rumor-monger, labors to connect confusions in the absence of totality, conclusion, and closure" (1995, 241). This leads to the question of how to write about violence, a question that was most thoroughly attended to by Veena Das in her work on India's Partition (Das 1995, 2007). As Das (1995) cautions, we should remain skeptical about our abilities to produce an account of violence on behalf of our interlocutors that does not distort their voices and distance us from their experiences. Writing about South Africa, Didier Fassin and colleagues (2008) highlight the difficulties of writing about violence that, especially for women, has many as-yet-uncovered dimensions. Both Das and Fassin and colleagues address the limitations of writing about violence by working with "fragments," which Das describes as "different from a part or various parts that may be assembled to make up a picture of totality. Unlike a sketch that may be executed on a different scale from the final picture one draws, or that may lack all the details of the picture but still contain the imagination of the whole, the fragment marks the impossibility of such an imagination" (Das 2007, 5). I return to the fragment in the book as a means of communicating participants' accounts of violence and how this powerful structuring force of how life is lived in Khayelitsha is at odds with the extended temporal horizon of the first 1,000 days.

OVERVIEW OF THE BOOK

Chapter 1 places the development of the concept of the first 1,000 days in the context of the interrelated histories of public health interventions in early life nutrition, epidemiological approaches to chronic disease, and understandings of heredity. Drawing on the anthropologies of postgenomics, the international and global health movements, and the future, the chapter demonstrates how the first 1,000 days has materialized as a specific object of global health concern and how South Africa has emerged as a key site of DOHaD science.

Chapter 2 situates this study in Khayelitsha and shows how the township is both a research hub on the global health map and a distinct site for understanding the intersections of colonial, apartheid, and post-apartheid histories; processes of urbanization; and the persistently racialized geographies of exclusion that characterize contemporary South Africa and its situated biologies.

In the third chapter, I attend to the question of how ideas about epigenetics and nutrition travel across policy and clinical domains in new biopolitical formations that authorize further incursions of state and nonstate actors into domestic spaces under the auspices of health care. Through ethnographic encounters in lecture theatres, international conferences, government offices and the homes of young women, I explore how Khayelitsha has become a central node in a broader research archipelago (Rottenburg 2009) where knowledge claims and policy around the first 1,000 days are forged and circulated. This chapter is about the location of potential in the archetypes of the mother-child dyad and the archipelago.

Chapter 4 takes the clinic as its primary ethnographic site and illustrates how nutrition policies are shaped, altered, navigated, and confounded by the material infrastructure of the clinics, staff improvisations amid huge patient loads and stock shortages, and the tensions between the policy prescriptions for individual behavior change and staff awareness of the constraints their patients face. In this chapter I document life between protocols, a space characterized by pragmatic forms of care and unknowing when it is impossible to extend such care. In this chapter I consider the complexities of the post-apartheid "neoliberal welfarist" state and who is responsible for the creation of potential and its realization.

Chapter 5 takes the ethnography into the homes and lives of women and their families in order to focus on the means by which people craft the future. While early life public health intervention increasingly turns on notions of intergenerational transmission, it is education, employment, entrepreneurship, and the navigation of bureaucracy and networks of kin that underline the securing of intergenerational well-being. The ethnography charts the uneven distribution of aspiration: some are able to make something out of nothing to work toward a desired future, but the future is much less certain for others. The chapter is about the disjuncture between the framing of potential in global health campaigns such as the first 1,000 days from the perspective of a distant future and the means by which ordinary people secure the present.

Whereas chapter 5 is concerned with aspiration, or the future in a representational sense, in chapter 6, I describe the affective dimensions of life lived in anticipation. I attend to the historical, social, and structural factors that shape maternal subjectivities and show how in a context of high levels of crime and violence, the anticipatory logic of a programmatic focus on maternal investment overlooks infrastructures of anticipation and their effects on intergenerational relations.

In the final chapter, I return to the book's central argument: that global health projects focused on the early life period are configured by a politics of potential that focuses intervention and situates responsibility in gendered, raced, and individualized bodies, and conceives of outcomes as something that will be achieved in the distant future, rather than as something that is currently within our grasp. I consider what this means for life and care in the particular configurations of state support in post-apartheid South Africa and I argue for caution in response to the continued expansion of global health attention to the category of early life.

1 · THE FIRST 1,000 DAYS

Origin Stories

"Go for the mother—she is the most important health care worker!" Published in the *South African Journal of Family Practice* in in a review article on interventions for protein-energy malnutrition (Bac and Glatthaar 1990), the advice to "go for the mother" illustrates the long-standing prominence of mothers as central figures in public health strategies. In writing their review, the authors—a clinician and a nutrition scientist—offered an expansive framing of protein-energy malnutrition as a "complex, sensitive problem which needs a multi-sectorial eco-logical approach" (284). Alongside the advice to focus on maternal education as part of a suite of primary health care strategies, the authors made recommenda-tions for the agricultural sector, the food industry, and the education sector and called for a host of socioeconomic and political interventions such as food subsi-dies, social support, water and sanitation, and the "abolition of restrictive and dis-criminatory legislation" (289).

The review, which was aimed at the community of primary health care practi-tioners in South Africa in the early 1990s, captures elements of the history into which first 1,000 days policies were enfolded some decades later, including a long-standing linkage between nutrition and maternal education; a continuing tussle between narrow, vertical interventions and a more expansive approach to preven-tion that includes considerations of food availability and food security; and a his-tory of colonial and apartheid laws that shaped the health profile of South Africa, referred to obliquely as "restrictive and discriminatory legislation."

In this chapter, I situate the first 1,000 days concept in these historical and material contexts. I start by considering three intersecting histories that formed the epistemological field for the emergence of a focus on the first 1,000 days: histories of the concept of heredity; epidemiological approaches to noncommu-nicable diseases; and public health interventions in perinatal nutrition. Thinking with the metaphor of gene-environment interactions, one might say that the his-tories I describe here constitute the milieu—that is, the conditions of possibility for the uptake of a set of concepts that inform contemporary ideas of health and life. In outlining these histories, I begin an archaeology of the first 1,000 days in the Foucauldian sense—an outline of "the systems of simultaneity, as well as the series of mutations necessary and sufficient to circumscribe the threshold of a new positivity" (Foucault 1970, xxiii). A review of the products of these milieus— genetic science, the international and global health movements, the future as imaginative horizon—reflects a genealogy of the place of biology in contemporary global health. In Michel Foucault's understanding, examining the genealogy of ideas allows for the tracing of the emergence of truths within contingent histories of power. In his 1984 lecture "What Is Enlightenment?" Foucault outlined both archaeology and genealogy as constitutive of what he calls historical ontology. This chapter is a historical ontology of the first 1,000 days and seeks to place particular histories of practice within a broader understanding of their conditions of possibility. Finally, I locate these histories within the specific context of South Africa.

THE FIRST 1,000 DAYS: SITUATED HISTORIES

First proposed in a *Lancet* series on maternal and child undernutrition (Bryce et al. 2008), the first 1,000 days concept has become a rallying point for international efforts against malnutrition. The *Lancet* review described the persistent global burden of undernutrition and recommended the integration of nutrition interventions with maternal and child health packages in thirty-six countries. The series focused on height for age at two years (roughly 1,000 days after conception) as the best predictor of future human capital, defined by adult height, educational achievement, future income, and the birth weight of future children (Victora et al. 2008). The use of these indices expresses the economic logic that underpins the first 1,000 days concept: good nutrition is a "prerequisite for economic development" (Bryce et al. 2008). In the same year, the UN secretary-general established the High-Level Task Force on Food and Nutrition Security and the Copenhagen Consensus concluded that nutrition was one of the most cost-effective investments for development (Copenhagen Consensus Center 2008). These events and recommendations later formed the basis for the UN's Scaling Up Nutrition program and the 1000 Days: Change a Life, Change the Future campaign. Using the 2008 *Lancet* series as a new evidence base for action and in line with the World Bank's shift to repositioning nutrition as central to development (World Bank 2006), Scaling Up Nutrition aimed to make nutrition a key concern for all sectors (United Nations 2010). The 1000 Days: Change a Life, Change the Future campaign was launched on September 21, 2010, by US secretary of state Hillary Clinton and Irish minister Micheál Martin at the UN General Assembly (Thurow 2016).

The *Lancet*'s follow-up series on maternal and child nutrition added that the first 1,000 days also impacts on potential future burdens of overnutrition and noncommunicable diseases (Black et al. 2013). As a key message, the 2013 series highlighted that "undernutrition during pregnancy, affecting fetal growth, and the first 2 years of life is a major determinant of both stunting of linear growth and subsequent obesity and non-communicable diseases in adulthood" (1). This set the scene for the first 1,000 days to become a key tool in the noncommunicable diseases prevention toolkit.

At the heart of the first 1,000 days concept is a revival of the nature/nurture debate and a disruption of what is understood as inherited and what is understood as acquired in contemporary biomedical understandings of health and disease outcomes. Therefore, a departure point for understanding the constitution of the first 1,000 days lies in the history of heredity, which emerged as an important concern for biology in the mid-nineteenth century. Until the late 1700s, the transmission of characteristics between parents and offspring was largely understood as part of *generation*, an Aristotelian view of development as gradual and sequential (Müller-Wille and Rheinberger 2012). The concept of biological inheritance—that something is transmitted from parent to progeny independent of developmental processes—was made prominent by Charles Darwin (1859) and Francis Galton (1869). From the nineteenth to the twenty-first centuries, the science of heredity cycled between hard and soft understandings of inheritance (Meloni 2016). In simplified terms, hard heredity refers to the notion that inheritance is fixed at conception and soft heredity understands hereditary material as malleable and shaped according to environmental factors (Meloni 2016, citing Bonduriansky 2012). Darwinian and Mendelian concepts of heredity are prominent examples of the former; Lamarckism most commonly represents the latter. In the 2000s, genetic determinism best represents the hard heredity argument and epigenetics exemplifies soft inheritance.

Philosopher of science Georges Canguilhem articulated this debate as one of a relationship between organism and milieu that has political implications: "Recognition of the milieu's determining action has a political social impact: it authorizes man's unlimited action on himself via the intermediary of the milieu" (Canguilhem 2008, 115). Thus, Canguilhem argued, the prevailing concept of heredity at any one time was as much dependent on its ideological underpinnings and political reception as on its scientific merit. In his analysis of changing social values in human heredity in the twentieth century, Maurizio Meloni termed this "political biology," the idea that knowledge claims must overcome "the constraints imposed by acceptable—that is to say, recognized—epistemic statements and available sociopolitical values" (Meloni 2016, 18). That new scientific ideas must find social acceptance to flourish partly explains why the field of epigenetics did not fully crystallize until the early twenty-first century, although a version of the concept of epigenetics has existed since the 1940s (Jablonka and Lamb 2002).

The histories of the fields of demography and public health are particularly interrelated with notions of hard heredity (Foucault 1976; Müller-Wille and

Rheinberger 2012). In the late nineteenth century, proponents of hard heredity, most prominently Galton, saw huge opportunity in enumerating population characteristics in order to improve the quality of a nation (Rose 2007). The eugenics movement that emerged in the first half of the twentieth century was characterized by a primacy of biology and scientific expertise, a utopian vision of future order, and the privileging of the population over the individual (Meloni 2016). Michel Foucault argued that this combination of the development of techniques of counting populations and the tight regulation of biological processes and heredity had its extreme expression in the Nazi regime. For Foucault (2003, 260), Nazi society illustrated "biopower in an absolute sense," and for many biopolitical thinkers, the Nazi eugenic logic continues to animate biopolitics in the present (see, e.g., Baumann 1989; Agamben 1998; Esposito 2008). Paul Rabinow and Nikolas Rose (2006) offer an alternative rendering of contemporary biopolitics as based on a logic of vitality brought forth in part by the molecularization of life processes. Drawing these philosophical debates into conversation with histories of heredity, Maurizio Meloni (2010) argues that Foucault did not intend for biopower or biopolitics to become ahistorical concepts and cautions against epochal views of biopower abstracted from specific historical and material contexts. Instead, he contends that an understanding of contemporary biopolitical forms requires a return to the Foucauldian method of locating ideas in specific and situated contexts, or what Foucault called historical ontology.

Several histories related to the first 1,000 days concept intersect with a history of ideas of heredity. The focus on the first 1,000 days has become popularized at a particular point in the history of heredity when a return to soft inheritance in the form of epigenetics is gaining currency. Closely related to this history, the first 1,000 days approach also represents the most recent manifestation of a series of shifts in epidemiological approaches to noncommunicable diseases toward incorporating life course perspectives over the course of the twentieth century. Finally, the first 1,000 days is one in a long line of interventions in maternal and child nutrition since the end of the nineteenth century that favor maternal education and behavioral interventions as the means of securing the social and economic benefits of population health, instead of adequate policy responses to the structural factors that shape food security and population well-being.

Heredity: The Return to Epigenetics

Maurizio Meloni (2016) cites two important factors after World War II that contributed to the consolidation of hard heredity as the dominant model in the second half of the twentieth century. First, the discovery of the structure of DNA by James Watson and Francis Crick (1953) and the nascent field of molecular biology offered a measurable biological basis for hard heredity. Advances in technology materialized the gene as a measurable object well before the same occurred for epigenetic phenomena (Müller-Wille and Rheinberger 2012). Second, postwar concepts of biological inheritance conformed to a universal rights–based ethos that emerged at that time (Haraway 1990). Genetics, a science that could celebrate individual difference, was compatible with notions of liberal democracy (Meloni 2016). Thus, although the gene was by no means a stable concept, by the end of the twentieth century it had been established as the dominant language of heredity (Fox Keller 2000). The Human Genome Project, which ran from 1990 to 2003 and sought to map the entire human genome, cemented the gene as central in popular understandings of heredity. However, the completion of the Human Genome Project led to far more complex understandings of the genome as a map of data in which the genotype is just one node among many in a complex systems network (Rheinberger 2013). Together with advances in information technology and mathematics, this led to a range of new approaches in systems biology and the collection of approaches referred to as the "omics" (Joyce and Palsson 2006).

Among the omics, epigenetics is described as the "archetypal postgenomic science" (Stevens and Richardson 2015, 4). Coined by Conrad Waddington in the 1940s, the term epigenetics derives from the Aristotelian concept of epigenesis, which emphasized the qualitative and continuous nature of development (Waddington 1942). Waddington (1968) wished to describe the biological study of the interaction between genes and their products, a possibility that would not manifest until later in the twentieth century with the expansion of the field of molecular biology. Understandings of epigenetics have changed with these advances (Jablonka and Lamb 2002) and controversy persists over the definition of the term (Ptashne 2007). One consensus definition of an epigenetic trait that has been proposed is "a stably heritable phenotype resulting from changes in a chromosome without alterations in the DNA sequence" (Berger et al. 2009, 781). A less technical definition describes epigenetics as "heritable changes in gene expression that cannot be tied to genetic variation" (Richards 2006, 396). What is clear is that definitions of epigenetics afford an ambiguity of use across a diverse set of concerns (Meloni and Testa 2014).

Knowledge of the processes by which epigenetic mechanisms interact with gene expression is still very limited (Landecker and Panofsky 2013). The best-described epigenetic phenomenon is DNA methylation, the process whereby marks on the epigenome manifest during development in response to environmental cues, among which nutritional signals are thought to be especially important (Waterland and Michels 2007). Less is known about other possible epigenetic mechanisms. This has not tempered excitement about the possibility of intergenerational transmission of disease risk, which has emerged as a powerful idea despite the paucity of evidence for transgenerational epigenetic inheritance in humans (Heard and Martienssen 2014). The two multigenerational studies most commonly cited in this case are the Dutch famine cohort (Roseboom et al. 2001) and the Swedish Överkalix cohort (Pembrey et al. 2006). In both the Netherlands and Sweden, meticulous health records were kept that allow for detailed retrospective analysis. The Dutch famine, the result of Nazi Germany's embargo on food supplies to the western Netherlands from October 1944 to May 1945, affected 4.5 million people. After exposure to famine in utero and early life, children born during this period demonstrated increased rates of obesity, metabolic disease, and other illnesses during adulthood, although this was dependent on several variables, including the timing of the exposure (Heijmans et al. 2008; Tobi et al. 2009). Researchers who assessed Överkalix parish registers for 1890, 1905, and 1920 also demonstrated a correlation between grandparental and parental nutrition in critical periods (measured by historical records of food prices and harvest success) with offspring risk of cardiovascular and metabolic disease (Kaati et al. 2002). This work showed sex-specific transmissions of mortality risk across two generations, again highlighting timing of exposure as an important factor (Pembrey et al. 2006). While scientists (Grossniklaus et al. 2013; Heard and Martienssen 2014) and social scientists (Meloni and Testa 2014; Pickersgill 2016) call for modesty in claims about the importance of transgenerational epigenetic inheritance, this idea has had a significant impact and the debate continues (Fitz-James and Cavalli 2022).

The role of epigenetic mechanisms in configuring disease outcomes has been of interest to social scientists, who have considered how DOHaD and epigenetics might provide explanatory mechanisms for health disparities and inequalities and a language for understanding the linkages between the biological and the social.[1] This research has also interrogated the expansion of epigenetics as a discourse in the scientific, social scientific, and public spheres, especially the figuring of the maternal body in epigenetic imaginaries, and has highlighted the positive political potential of epigenetic discourses for opening up understandings of bodies and environments as plastic entities, versus the negative possibilities of reconstituted forms of biological determinism.[2]

Although advances in genome studies have generated hype around the prospects of personalized medicine, pharmacogenomics and genome sequencing has so far had only limited application in clinical settings. Epigenetics and omics research introduce unwieldy complexities for modeling population health. As epidemiologist and science studies scholar Susanne Bauer has noted, integrating epigenomic variables and their many interactions into epidemiological models "pushes the limits of statistical validity" (Bauer 2013, 523). Using largely molecular variables "folds individual and population into each other," which has challenging implications for the application of epidemiological findings (525). For example, mapping the exposome—the sum total of exposures that might impact on disease risk across the life course (Wild 2005)—is a daunting if not impossible task for epidemiology (DeBord et al. 2016). The need to manage such complexity is one reason for epidemiologists to focus on stages of the life course thought to play a more critical role in shaping future disease risk, including adolescence and early life (Ben-Shlomo et al. 2016). In sum, even while there is still much to learn about epigenetics, these shifting notions of inheritance and disease risk have had a significant impact on epidemiological theory and practice.

Histories of Epidemiology: Noncommunicable Diseases, the Life Course, and DOHaD

The evolution of epidemiological ideas about noncommunicable diseases in the twentieth and twenty-first centuries and more specifically the formalization of the field of DOHaD research is also important for understanding the emergence of the first 1,000 days concept. Starting in the 1800s, the field of epidemiology assembled the possibilities of scientific and statistical advances for describing and enumerating diseases and disease patterns (Foucault 2008; Latour 1988). Debates about heredity, statistical and medical studies of mortality patterns, and public health programs in the late nineteenth and early twentieth centuries closely informed each other (Kuh and Davey Smith 1993). For example, concerns about the fitness of British men to serve in the Anglo-Boer War in South Africa (1899–1902) led to government interest in the physical health of the nation and thus to interest in adult and infant mortality rates. As historian Anna Davin notes, investment in infant well-being became of "imperial importance" (1978, 14).

Around the same time, proponents of eugenics, such as Galton's student Karl Pearson, argued that infant mortality was another expression of natural selection that prevented the development of weak "stock" (Kuh and Smith 1993). Early twentieth-century epidemiology was characterized by attempts to understand the relationship between patterns of disease, hereditary factors, and the influence of social and environmental conditions. The latter gave rise to the field of occupational health. One important focus of this period was early life as a time that could affect adult "vitality" (Kermack et al. 1934).

In her comprehensive analysis of the evolution of epidemiology in the twentieth century, social epidemiologist Nancy Krieger (2011) shows how the discipline shifted from a focus on germs and genes in the first half of the century to the risk factor and lifestyle models that dominated after the 1960s. Improved computational methods in the 1950s made possible the testing of multifactorial hypotheses (Susser 1985), and epidemiologists expanded their frameworks of agent, host, and environment to include a range of factors that could contribute to ill health, often captured in the shorthand term "lifestyle" (Krieger 2011). The first large cohort study of its kind, the Framingham study on coronary heart disease (Dawber and Kannel 1958), embodied this new approach, and out of this work emerged a new focus for epidemiological attention: "the risk factor" (Kannel et al. 1961). Cohort analysis became a key epidemiological methodology for studying the relationship between risk factors and outcomes for disease in adult life (Kuh and Davey Smith 1993). The post–World War II discipline of chronic disease epidemiology was concerned with statistically measurable proximate exposures and outcomes rather than with early life associations (Saracci 2007) and the postwar focus on environmental or "lifestyle" exposures in adulthood supplanted the early-twentieth-century public health concern with early life influences on chronic diseases and mortality risk. That focus reemerged in the 1970s as the concept of developmental programming gained currency (Kuh and Davey Smith 1993).

Developmental programming theory demonstrated the predictive role of poor conditions in early life for possible adult disease. Several studies of the 1970s and 1980s challenged prevailing understandings of the etiology of noncommunicable diseases (Dörner 1973; Forsdahl 1977; Wadsworth et al. 1985; Notkola et al. 1985). The term "programming" is attributed to Dörner (1973), who noted an association between perinatal conditions and risk for adult atherosclerosis and obesity and advocated for improved maternal care in East Germany (Dörner et al. 2008). Freinkel (1980) later postulated that maternal metabolic function influences the development of fetal structures with long-term effects. However, the origin story of DOHaD is most often traced to the work of David Barker and Clive Osmond (1986), whose research on the association of poor childhood nutrition and adult cardiovascular diseases in deprived English counties produced the thrifty phenotype (or fetal origins) hypothesis.[3] This hypothesis contends that conditions during critical windows of development have a long-term effect on function or morphology (Hales and Barker 1992). These ideas supported the return of the "critical period" as a key concept in life course epidemiology, defined as "a limited time window in which an exposure can have adverse or protective effects on development and subsequent disease outcome" (Kuh et al. 2003). Critics of developmental programming theory highlighted the difficulties of proving causality given the long gap between exposure and outcome and dismissed observations as ecological associations (Joseph and Kramer 1996). Others observed that the critical period of development is ill defined (Ulijaszek 1996). Nevertheless, animal models and epidemiological studies in many settings display the correlations that developmental programming theory suggests (Delisle 2002). By the late 1990s, the establishment of life course epidemiology as a distinct field dovetailed with the formalization of DOHaD as an established research field with its own journals and professional associations (Richardson 2015; Ben-Shlomo et al. 2016).

In the twenty-first century, epigenetics has provided substantive methods for measuring exposure and outcome beyond the correlational tools that have provided evidence for developmental programming. DOHaD researchers have readily embraced the language of epigenetics as a way of describing intergenerational models of disease distribution. The first 1,000 days concept is one expression of this logic and the most recent in a long line of policy interventions in perinatal nutrition.

Public Health Approaches to Perinatal Nutrition

My intention here is not to offer a definitive account of the history of public health approaches to perinatal nutrition but to highlight the aspects that are important to understanding the present-day focus on early life. Nutrition in early life was a key focus of early twentieth-century concerns with improving adult "vitality" and an impetus for programs that addressed the welfare of mothers and children (Davin 1978; Kuh and Smith 1993). The relationship between diet and health became strategically important for the aspirations of Euro-American nations seeking a "fit stock" of workers and soldiers. As Anson Rabinbach (1990) describes, the relationship between work, fatigue, and nutrition emerged as a concern for European scientists in the late nineteenth century. Public health interventions frequently focused on the maternal-child dyad, often naturalizing the mother as the primary caregiver (Wheeler 1985; Baird 2008) and the child as a signifier of innocence and potentiality (Castañeda 2002). The tropes of the "ignorant mother" and the "innocent child" in nutrition interventions persisted throughout the twentieth century.

The increased state interest in the regulation of population health buoyed maternal and child welfare programs from the early twentieth century until the end of World War II in industrialized nations and their colonies. In 1904, a *British Medical Journal* editorial concluded that "it cannot be too often repeated that a child wisely fed for the first two or three years of life has every chance of growing into a strong man or woman; a child rendered rickety and puny by ignorant feeding will in all probability never make up the ground it has lost" (quoted in Dwork 1987). Maternal education was an early focus of nutrition programs, and a new science of motherhood emerged alongside nutrition science in the United States (Apple 1987) and the United Kingdom (Smith 1997). In African contexts, maternal and child health programs in the first half of the twentieth century exemplified the focus on "nutritional science" and privileged infant welfare over maternal health (Vaughan 1988). As historian Megan Vaughan (1988, 132) explains, scientists in the 1930s held the view "that nutrition was the key to ill health in Africa, and that nutritional science, harnessing the skills of the anthropologists, had a major role to play in improving the health status of African peoples." Audrey Richards' (1939) classic study of the Bemba is one such outcome of research funded for the purpose of investigating nutrition in the colonies. She showed that child malnutrition in this setting was a product of social and economic circumstances, and not due to the ignorance of African women, which was the prevailing notion at the time (1939).

After World War II, institutions were established to steer a program of international development that would see all countries achieve a Western ideal of prosperity and progress. A key international development project of the latter half of the twentieth century was the eradication of hunger and malnutrition, which was formalized with the formation of the UN's Food and Agriculture Organization in 1945. Another was the provision of universal health care, which was formalized with the formation of the UN's World Health Organization in 1948 and was later embodied in the Alma Ata Declaration of 1978.[4] The comprehensive primary health care package that Alma Ata espoused was only partially implemented in the form of selective primary health care programs (Rifkin and Walt 1986). For pragmatic and political reasons, women and children were often the focus of these interventions, which were geared largely toward the dual problems of undernutrition and infection (Scrimshaw et al. 1959, 1968). The best example is UNICEF's widespread rollout of its GOBI-FFF strategy in the 1980s, which at first included growth monitoring, oral rehydration, breastfeeding, and immunization (GOBI) and was later expanded to include family planning, female education, and food supplementation (FFF), especially during pregnancy.[5] The success of the GOBI program rested on its "low-cost, high-impact" nature, foreshadowing the shift in focus in the 1980s and 1990s to a market-based logic for health care interventions that would be efficient and cost effective (Basilico et al. 2013, 82).

A key figure for postwar development interventions was the "marasmic [undernourished] child in its mother's arms"—an iconic image of a vulnerable child in need of the developed world's aid (Wheeler 1985, 133; Burman 1994). Nutritionist Erica Wheeler (1985) questioned the frequently deployed concept of "vulnerable groups" to describe children and pregnant and lactating women. While she concurred that these were periods of physiological vulnerability, she disagreed with the policy emphasis on maternal nutrition education, which translated into a model in which "access to a good diet is limited by the woman's knowledge and skills" and "the 'vulnerable' young child is the first to suffer" (476). Wheeler argued that nutrition programs that focused solely on maternal education translated to maternal blame because they assumed that "a mother whose child is malnourished, if she has been subjected to health or nutrition education, must have refused to practice what she has learnt" (139). It is telling that some twenty years after Wheeler's critique, Devi Sridhar's (2008) ethnography of a World Bank nutrition program revealed that the same assumptions underpinned the international focus on maternal nutrition education: mothers are the sole caregivers, they have decision-making power, and child undernutrition can be alleviated through education to correct "feminized, ignorant and backward" beliefs (78). Here again, the aim was to influence maternal behavior on the basis that undernutrition was the result of poor maternal practices that could be improved with education. This is despite the long-standing work that has demonstrated the complexity of the relationship between gender and food security and that maternal education alone is insufficient without also addressing equality in the labor force, equality in purchasing power, and equality of food distribution in households (Njuki et al. 2016).

The figuration of the "good mother" has also been prominent in debates about infant feeding. While debates about the perils of infant formula trace back to the 1920s (Manderson 1982), the 1974 court case between Nestlé and the Third World Action Group following its publication of a pamphlet entitled *Nestlé Kills Babies* is considered a seminal moment in the history of advocacy for breastfeeding (Van Esterik 2013). Researchers in the early 1970s had pointed to the rise in malnutrition and infection that accompanied the use of formula (Jeliffe 1972). The work of advocacy groups in the 1970s and 1980s led to the World Health Assembly's adoption of the International Code of Marketing of Breast-milk Substitutes in 1981. Following the discovery that HIV may be transmitted in breast milk (Ziegler et al. 1985), policy recommendations were revised for HIV-positive mothers, who were initially advised not to breastfeed. These policies were revised again after research showed that exclusive breastfeeding carried a much lower risk of HIV transmission than mixed feeding (the addition of water, formula, or other fluids or foods that might injure an infant's gastrointestinal mucosa) (Coutsoudis et al. 1999). Anthropologists have chronicled the effects of the global distribution of commercial infant formula (Scheper-Hughes 1984), the subsequent policy move by the World Health Organization and other international organizations to endorse exclusive breastfeeding (Gottshang 2000; Castro and Marchand-Lucas 2000), and controversies surrounding infant feeding in the context of HIV (Leshabari et al. 2007; Moland and Blystad 2009; van Hollen 2011). Across this literature, the "good mother" makes her feeding choice based on medico-scientific risk calculations (Murphy 2000). The implications, again, are that women's breasts and bodies are "risky environments" (Van Esterik 2002, 272): mothers are responsible for infant health and, in the case of HIV, infants' HIV-negative status and survival (Moland and Blystad 2009; Fassin 2013).

The prioritization of nutrition and the health and well-being of women and children persisted into the 2000s in five of the UN's eight Millennium Development Goals.[6] These goals functioned as a spearheading mechanism in the formation of the public-private partnerships that characterize the contemporary global health landscape. For key donors such as the Bill & Melinda Gates Foundation, maternal and child health and nutrition continues to be an important focus. Launched in 2000, the Global Alliance for Vaccines and Immunization, funded by the Gates Foundation, continues the work of the GOBI program, albeit with a narrower mandate of targeted interventions (Basilico et al. 2013).

The first 1,000 days campaign is thus a present-day articulation of the initial public health approach of the late 1900s, based on the premise that early life nutrition governs both present and future health, now newly constituted as a life course epidemiology approach to preventing noncommunicable diseases. The infographic produced by the NGO 1,000 Days (Figure 2) captures the promise of this renewed focus on the early life period: "the impact of nutrition in

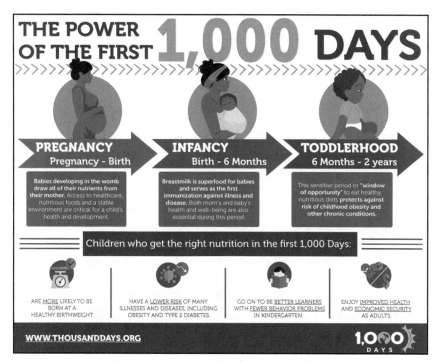

FIGURE 2. First 1,000 Days program infographic. (Source: www.thousanddays.org. © 1,000 Days)

early life can reach far into the future" to impact disease risk, cognitive development, and future earning potential.[7]

In South Africa, the implementation of first 1,000 days policies is inflected by the particular histories of perinatal nutrition in this context, including attitudes toward maternal and child welfare in the colonial and apartheid eras and the role of infant feeding in the country's public health response to the HIV epidemic.

PERINATAL NUTRITION IN SOUTH AFRICA

The history of perinatal nutrition interventions in South Africa has been profoundly shaped by the country's colonial and apartheid past. Dutch (1652–1800) and then British (1800–1910) colonialism established public health legislation and biomedical hospital care in South Africa. Christian missionaries played a significant role in importing British models of "respectable motherhood" in the early twentieth century (Gaitskell 1992; Burns 1995). From 1910 to 1948, progressive advocacy for a unified national health service was based on a primary health care model, and South Africa is thus often credited as the birthplace of social medicine (Kautszky and Tollman 2008). One of the origins of the primary health care model is the Pholela Health Centre, established in rural Natal in 1940 by Sidney and Emily Kark.[8] The comprehensive Pholela model integrated curative and preventive care and provided health education and health promotion. The center placed health in a framework of family, community, and social determinants that was profoundly progressive for the time (Kautzky and Tollman 2008). The Pholela model was influential in the National Health Services Commission in 1942, which resulted in the Gluckman Report of 1944, which promoted a national health system that was not dissimilar to the system that would develop in the United Kingdom. However, the report and its recommendations for planned innovative health care and nutrition policies were abandoned after the ratification of apartheid policies in 1948 (Marks and Andersson 1992).

Apartheid was a system of legislated racial segregation and discrimination in South Africa from 1948 until the first democratic elections in 1994.[9] Understandings of heredity and potential are historically inflected in South Africa by long-standing forms of scientific racism. Historian Saul Dubow (1995) has demonstrated the close relationship between the formalization of apartheid and shifting notions of heredity and race in the postwar era. In the 1930s, Afrikaner nationalism invoked Nazi ideologies of White supremacy and racial purity. After World War II, these ideas became politically unpalatable. They also failed to explain the heterogeneity of White society in South Africa and the phenomenon of "poor whites" (Dubow 1995, 166). After World War II, the founders of apartheid used a development thesis to justify legislation to segregate races so that "different groups" could develop according to their own prescribed "stages of development" and according to their own potential (Dubow 1995). As James Scott describes it, the apartheid project was premised on an "authoritarian high modernism" that justified "separate development" policies based on racial classification (Scott 1998, 89). Although decolonization projects unfolded elsewhere in Africa in the 1950s, in South Africa the rhetoric of decolonization was used to rationalize the creation of independent bantustans and the state sought to relinquish responsibility for the welfare of "homeland" citizens (Wylie 2001).[10]

The apartheid government's approach to health and nutrition in the 1950s was based on a paternalistic notion of an "ignorant, non-scientific Africa" (Wylie 2001, 234). In the 1960s, South African nutrition science contributed to international research on protein-energy malnutrition (kwashiorkor) and the government instituted milk and cereal distribution programs in line with UNICEF recommendations. However, these schemes and the recording of statistics were abandoned in 1968 as part of a wider state denial of African hunger. In the 1970s, the state adopted the primary health care language of the international health community, but as eminent South African pediatrician Hoosen Coovadia (1988) noted, this was merely an appropriation of the terms with no meaningful outcomes. A fragmented, grassroots primary health care movement delivered initiatives such as GOBI-FFF in South Africa in the 1980s (Kuhn et al. 1990; den Besten et al. 1995; Kautzky and Tollman 2008). As in the review article mentioned at the beginning of this chapter, mothers were a core focus of primary health care strategies. This was also evident in training textbooks for health care workers in the early 1990s. The *Manual of Community Nursing and Communicable Diseases: A Textbook for South African Students* stated that "unenlightened mothers do not comprehend the need for prevention" (Vlok 1991, 402) and advocated for a primary health care approach with a strong focus on the health education of the mother, for example in "housecrafts and the cooking of nutritious meals for the family" (35).

In 1994, the first nationally representative nutrition study on children below 6 years of age showed that one in four South African children was stunted and that there was a high prevalence of micronutrient deficiencies in that age group (South African Vitamin A Consultative Group 1995). That year, the new democratic government rolled out the Integrated Nutrition Program, which had a significant and sustained focus on maternal and child nutrition (Department of Health 1998). Rising obesity rates in Black South Africans were first noted in a 1998 national survey, which showed that 25.4 percent of Black African men and 58.5 percent of Black African women were overweight or obese (Puoane et al. 2002). Subsequent surveys in 2003, 2009, and 2013 showed an upward trend and a persistently increased risk of obesity in Black African women compared to other groups.[11] The South African Nutrition and Health Survey of 2013 showed that childhood stunting had increased in the 0–3 year age group and had decreased slightly in older age groups. In addition, rates of overweight and obesity in adults and children had risen rapidly (Shisana et al. 2013). The turn to a focus on early life nutrition for both child and adult health outcomes is clear in the survey's recommendations that the combination of the pattern of childhood stunting and rising obesity rates warranted interventions "during and even before pregnancy, as well as during the important 'window of opportunity' up to around two years of age" (Shisana et al. 2013, 212).

Studying Transitions

Before democracy, obesity in Black Africans attracted little interest, partly because of a theory that Black Africans developed "healthy or benign obesity" (Walker et al. 1989). This concept prevailed until at least the early 2000s (Walker et al. 2001) despite extensive work that refutes it (Levitt et al. 1993; Kruger et al. 2001). After the "benign obesity" hypothesis was discredited, South African scientists showed significant interest in the "ethnic" differences in the manifestation of obesity and metabolic disease. Research comparing the metabolisms and anthropometry of racial groups (using South African census categories) suggested differences in levels of insulin resistance (Van der Merwe et al. 2000), hormone levels (Buthulezi et al. 2000), and visceral fat (Punyadeera et al. 2001), among others (Kruger et al. 2005, Van der Merwe et al. 2006). South African biomedicine and nutrition science in the early years of democracy thus appears to have perpetuated conflations of race and genetics, citing "ethnic variability" as a common explanation for differences in racial health outcomes. However, genetic and "ethnic" explanations for rising rates of obesity and noncommunicable diseases in South Africa have been much less prominent than epidemiological explanations that have cited urbanization and concomitant dietary and lifestyle change as key drivers of obesity and noncommunicable diseases.

Since the late 1990s, theories of nutrition transition have dominated epidemiological framings of obesity, diabetes, and cardiovascular disease in South Africa.[12] Nutrition transition is a concept developed by Barry Popkin (1993) as an extension of theories of demographic (Thompson 1929; Caldwell 1976) and epidemiological (Omran 1971) transitions to illustrate how diet and energy expenditure and their correlating disease states have shifted in concert with population and economic changes. Epidemiologists have ascribed differences in the health outcomes of racial groups in South Africa in the apartheid period to separate epidemiological transitions: a "First World" pattern among Whites and a "Third World" transition among Black Africans that was expected to shift to a "First World" picture as urbanization unfolded (Myer et al. 2004). South Africa's national nutrition profile is also said to exemplify the "protracted-polarized" model of epidemiological transition (Frenk et al. 1989), which is characterized by a dual burden of obesity and undernutrition at the national, community and even household level.

The concept of transition has particular salience in South Africa as a framework for understanding political processes as well as changes in demography and population health. In the late 1980s, after decades when the apartheid government did not record any data on the health and nutrition of Black Africans, biologist Noel Cameron, then based at the University of the Witwatersrand, wrote a letter to Andries Brink, then president of the South African Medical Research Council. He argued that research on human growth was fundamental for understanding child health during what was likely to be a period of massive sociopolitical change in South Africa (Radin and Cameron 2012). To Cameron's surprise, Brink requested a meeting with him and introduced him to Medical Research Council epidemiologist Derek Yach. In 1990, the council funded the initiation of a birth cohort in Soweto, Johannesburg, to study the questions Cameron had posed about child and adult health during a period of significant transition in South Africa. Initially called the Birth to Ten Cohort, the Soweto cohort is now the Birth to Thirty Cohort (Richter et al. 2007; Richter 2022). It has provided the first longitudinal picture of child, adolescent, and adult health in South Africa. Along with the Pelotas Birth Cohort Study (Brazil), the Institute of Nutrition of Central America and Panama Nutrition Trial Cohort (Guatemala), the New Delhi Birth Cohort (India), and the Cebu Longitudinal Health and Nutrition Survey cohort (Philippines), Birth to Thirty is part of the Consortium of Health-Orientated Research in Transitioning Societies (Richter et al. 2012).

As the consortium's title suggests, an important commonality across the five sites is that they are thought to be undergoing transition. DOHaD scientists posit that economic and nutrition transition sets up the conditions that confer lifetime risk for adult noncommunicable diseases (Godfrey et al. 2010). They theorize that in contexts where food scarcity and undernutrition may have been prevalent, undernourished mothers give birth to infants who are metabolically geared for an environment of restricted nutrition (an evolutionary adaptation). As the nutrition transition unfolds and calorie-dense food becomes available, this generation experiences "environmental mismatch" and develops obesity and noncommunicable diseases (Gluckman and Hanson 2006). Maternal diabetes and obesity in this second generation are thought to predict the same conditions in their offspring via overnutrition pathways (Gluckman et al. 2010). The historical and present nutritional profiles of Brazil, Guatemala, the Philippines, India, and South Africa have in common this suggested transition and its attendant effects on population health. Most important for the story of the first 1,000 days, these five cohorts informed the 2008 *Lancet* series on maternal and child undernutrition, and interventions to correct overnutrition or undernutrition in pregnancy and early childhood have since been framed as especially relevant for nations thought to be undergoing nutrition transition.

THE FIRST 1,000 DAYS IN SOUTH AFRICA

Traditional models of energy balance are inadequate to explain the surge in obesity and "chronic diseases of lifestyle" in South Africa. However, DOHaD theories have proved a neat fit (Levitt et al. 2002) and have been met with much enthusiasm as a framework for "steering" the nutrition transition "in a more positive direction" (Vorster et al. 2011; Reddy and Mbewu 2016).

Since 2013, a focus on the first 1,000 days to alleviate both child undernutrition and adult obesity and noncommunicable diseases has informed South Africa's National Nutrition Policy, an outcome of collaboration between the Nutrition Directorate of South Africa's Department of Health, UNICEF, World Health Organization regional affiliates, and the Global Alliance for Improved Nutrition (Department of Health 2013a). While this policy is modeled on the UN's 2010 Road Map to Scale Up Nutrition, South Africa has never formally joined the Scaling Up Nutrition network. Commenting after the African Nutrition Congress in Bloemfontein in 2012, Lawrence Haddad (2012), executive director of the Global Alliance for Improved Nutrition and a prominent figure in international development, speculated that this could be because South Africa wished to avoid certain donors and the formal chains of accountability that membership in the network includes. Another account cited the research director at the Division of Human Nutrition at Stellenbosch University, Milla McLachlan, who questioned "devoting very limited senior nutrition capacity to a slow-to-take-off initiative versus getting it on the National Development Plan agenda" (IRIN 2012).[13] The uptake of the first 1,000 days concept in South African nutrition policy was thus not a case of straightforward translation from international frameworks. Stakeholders and partnerships were subject to their own distinct sets of regional politics and it traversed its way into policy via other channels.

Focused on the first 1,000 days, the 2013 National Nutrition Policy targeted a majority of interventions toward infants, children, and pregnant and lactating women. These included a therapeutic feeding scheme for the treatment of moderate to severe child undernutrition, a micronutrient and deworming program for children, therapeutic intervention for undernutrition in pregnancy, and interventions designed to change maternal behavior. The latter included the promotion of exclusive breastfeeding, education on complementary feeds, and education about "healthy eating for optimal weight management" during pregnancy and lactation (Department of Health 2013a, 19). An important outcome of this policy document was that it integrated nutrition, which previously had been the purview of social welfare, into maternal and child health services. In practice, this translated into the inclusion of mid-upper arm circumference (MUAC) and body mass index (BMI) measurements at a woman's first antenatal visit. BMI is calculated by dividing weight by the square of a person's height. A BMI of less than 18.5 is classified as undernutrition and a BMI of greater than 30 is classified as obesity. The MUAC is measured at the midpoint between the tip of the shoulder and the tip of the elbow using a tape measure with the arm hanging freely and the elbow extended. A MUAC of less than 23 centimeters indicates undernutrition; more than 33 centimeters indicates obesity (Department of Health 2015). According to the 2013 policy, if the MUAC and BMI measurements indicate undernutrition according to protocol criteria, then a woman should be referred to a therapeutic nutrition program; if she is of "normal" weight or overweight, she should receive nutrition and lifestyle modification counseling.

In the Western Cape, the nutrition policy and the first 1,000 days approach are part of the policy goals of the publication *Healthcare 2030: The Road to Wellness* (Western Cape Government Health 2014). These policies exemplify the politics of potential: policy achievements are made via a focus on particular bodies, they focus on individual responsibility, and they are part of a future horizon of progress. Both national and provincial policies are focused on a rights-based approach, the empowerment of citizens, and maximizing potential. They adopt a life course approach "in keeping with the prioritization of the 1,000 days of life which has a huge impact on the life of the child and the mother" (24). The Western Cape's policy defines wellness as "not merely the absence of disease but the ability to maximize personal potential in all spheres of life . . . not a state of being but a proactive process of increasing knowledge and agency for making healthier lifestyle choices and for adapting to changing circumstances towards realizing, maximizing and mobilizing the fullest potential" (15).

These recommendations are made against the backdrop of a controversial history of nutrition and antenatal and infant feeding policies in the context of HIV exposure in South Africa. Pregnant women—the first recipients of state-provided antiretrovirals for the prevention of mother-to-child transmission—were at the heart of debates about improving nutrition versus providing antiretrovirals (Labadarios et al. 2005; Burton et al. 2015; Fassin 2007; Cousins 2015). Mothers emerged as blameworthy targets in a powerful rhetoric of "children as victims" (Fassin 2013) and nowhere was debate more charged than in the context of infant feeding. Policies about infant feeding in South Africa have changed several times since the 2000s.[14] From 2002 to 2011, the national policy included both exclusive breastfeeding and exclusive formula feeding as options for the first six months of an infant's life and the government provided free formula to HIV-positive women who chose exclusive formula feeding. In 2011, the national policy shifted to follow the World Health Organization's 2010 guidelines and adopted the Tswhane Declaration of Support for Breastfeeding in South Africa, which advises all women to breastfeed exclusively for six months and to continue to breastfeed for at least one year regardless of maternal HIV status (Department of Health 2013b). When Kwazulu-Natal Province was the first to discontinue free formula distribution in 2011, the local responses were ambivalent (Ijumba et al. 2013). In 2014, the Western Cape province was the last to stop formula distribution.

The first 1,000 days project thus converges with a complex history of state and individual rights and responsibilities that crystallized during the HIV pandemic in democratic South Africa. The history of HIV interventions is central to the history of global health in Africa. The next chapter turns to Khayelitsha, a key site in that history, where some of the first HIV antiretroviral pilot programs were rolled out in 1999 as a coordinated effort among Médecins Sans Frontières, the Treatment Action Campaign, and the School of Family Medicine and Public Health at the University of Cape Town. The Khayelitsha pilot programs were crucial in demonstrating that provision of antiretrovirals was feasible on a large scale, and they were the forerunners to the rollout of antiretrovirals in the South African public sector. Khayelitsha is thus a particularly important site for understanding how the practice of government by exception that the HIV/AIDS crisis legitimized in Africa (Nguyen 2009) has given way to global health interventions in ordinary domains of primary care.

2 · SITUATED BIOLOGIES
The View from Khayelitsha

Early life interventions informed by a first 1,000 days logic rely on an epigenetic configuration of the pregnant body as "environment." Studying such an intervention in context thus invites a question: If mothers are foregrounded (Pentecost and Ross 2019), what is in the background? What does the boundary work of a maternal focus exclude from view? As postcolonial and feminist science and technology studies scholars have shown, "capital, labor, time, geography and scale" all require close attention if we are to situate and understand the specific events of any one technological intervention (Roy 2018, 49). A study of the rollout of perinatal nutrition policy focused on the first 1,000 days in Khayelitsha, Cape Town, is thus also a study of intersecting axes, including colonial, apartheid, and post-apartheid histories; trajectories of urbanization and development; and racialized and gendered labor and capital in the colony and postcolony.

In this chapter, I attend to multiple vantage points that illustrate Khayelitsha's place in a larger spatiotemporal network, including its geological and geomorphological characteristics and the history and political economy of the region, to decenter the usual valences of Khayelitsha in the urban imaginary of Cape Town and to offer a detailed account of the elements that shape the situated biologies of this place.

CARTOGRAPHIC IMAGINATIONS

Spanning forty square kilometers, Khayelitsha is bordered in the west by Mitchell's Plain; in the southeast by the R310 freeway, Monwabisi Beach, and the Indian Ocean; and in the north by the N2 highway (Figure 3).[1] Built on nonarable land, Khayelitsha is a series of sandy dunes surrounded by wetlands that are the result of erosion of the middle of the Table Mountain Sandstone formation that dominates the geology and geomorphology of the Western Cape. Khayelitsha thus lies on the most recent geological stratum of the Cape Peninsula, the

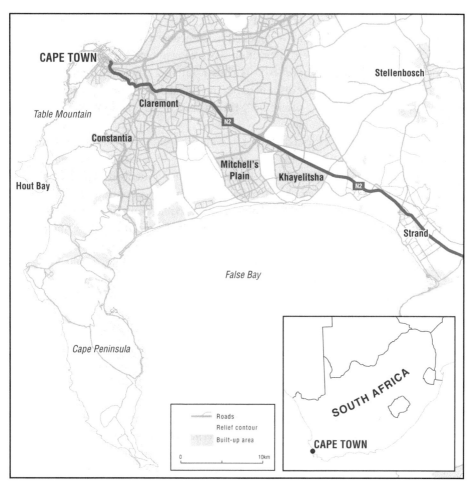

FIGURE 3. Map of Cape Town highlighting Khayelitsha in relation to other sites and the N2 highway. (Map by Miles Irving)

product of river-, sea-, and wind-derived sediments that formed the calcareous dunes of the Cape Flats (Holmes and Meadows 2012).

Some describe life in the informal settlements of Khayelitsha as life "characterized by absence—the absence of formal housing, the absence of employment, and the absence of infrastructure" (Storey 2014, 407). Entering Khayelitsha, one will immediately notice that the edges of the township are grazing grounds for livestock: cattle and goats are herded around the grassy wetlands between the highway and the start of dense rows of zinc shanties and concrete toilet blocks in various states of disrepair. Many residents have individual satellite dishes and are connected to a maze of power lines, but those who cannot afford electricity or who are not connected to the grid illegally siphon electricity from neighboring areas via cables that run through the sand (Mills 2016). By contrast, in established parts of Khayelitsha, such as Ilitha Park, brick houses are painted in pastel or bright colors and addresses are stenciled in curlicues across the façade. Here, building rubble signals the construction work of residents with the means to upgrade their homes. Khayelitsha is thus a far more heterogenous space than academic and popular discourse portrays, which tends to represent it as a homogenous place ("the township") that is fixed in time and inhabited by a homogenous group of people.

As one government official described it to me, Khayelitsha is both "magical and tragic." This contrasting narrative appears frequently in academic, government, and public accounts of Khayelitsha. For example, it is described as a township marked by poverty and unemployment but one "with its eyes on the future" (Cape Town Tourism 2015) and as both a "previously deprived locality" and an "investment destination" (Ngxiza 2012, 185). It is "in, but not of Cape Town" (Du Toit and Neves 2007, 18); a place that "both captivates and appalls" (MacGregor 2003, 2).

As well meaning as these contradictory descriptions might be, their effect is to flatten rather than illuminate complexity and to repeat a distancing and displacement of Khayelitsha from Cape Town. Against the common juxtaposition of city and township, Khayelitsha is much better understood as a node in a wide set of rural-urban circulations (Spiegel 1996). The "politics of density" (Murphy 2018, 119) particular to Cape Town index a distribution of violence in the city that is disproportionately borne by the residents of the city's townships (Pentecost and Cousins 2017). As anthropologist Kelly Gillespie (2014) explains, "The township is reinscribed as a separate place, excluded from the imaginations of the city proper, continuously peripheralized. The kind of life that occurs in the township is imagined to emerge *sui generis* from the township 'itself'. And the problems that arise in the township are understood to be problems that must be fixed *inside* the township" (210). Famously captured in Neill Blomkamp's 2009 film *District 9*, the township is an alien place, a trope that repeats across research, media, and public platforms as if there were "one giant citizen roaming around there" (Mqombothi 2014). In a dominant urban imaginary, Cape Town and Khayelitsha are configured as "*not the same place*," a slippage that denies recognition of the township as produced by and integral to the city (Gillespie 2014, 206, emphasis in original).

In this imaginary, these separate places are linked only by the N2 highway— Khayelitsha's access route to Cape Town's central business district. A notoriously dangerous road and a site of frequent protests, the N2 looms large in the cartographic imagination of city and township and figures prominently in work on Khayelitsha (Makhulu 2010; Robins 2014). Geographers Stanley Brunn and Matthew Wilson (2013) observe that this highway is the only experience of Khayelitsha that some Capetonians have ever had—a glimpse of government housing and closely built shacks behind the concrete-pillar barrier that separates the township from the road. The N2 connects the "series of islands" that constitute

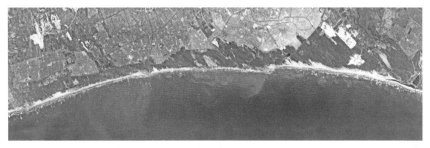

FIGURE 4. *False Bay #1*. (Photograph by Vincent Bezuidenhout, 2011. Used with permission)

Cape Town: some are high-end tourist destinations and others have "services and facilities barely fit for human beings" (Mlungwana and Kramer 2019, 9). As Brunn and Wilson contend, in this frame, Khayelitsha is Cape Town's terra incognita: unmapped in terms of both its incomplete cartography and its exclusion from a cosmopolitan Capetonian social landscape. Their assessment of sources that include aerial photographs, Google Maps, Google Street View, and digital placemarks highlights the incomplete mapping of the township—the uneven naming of streets and the poor coverage of Khayelitsha in Google Maps beyond major roads. Their analysis of Google search results, Google Scholar, and travel sites also shows how Khayelitsha is narrowly mapped in terms of cultural geography; few sources offer anything beyond a standard narrative of the township as one of Cape Town's poorest urban centers. They argue for expanding the cartographic imaginary of Khayelitsha—a task for geographers, social scientists, journalists, and artists.

One way to decenter the dominant view of Khayelitsha is to look toward the ocean. Khayelitsha is coastal. While the Indian Ocean bears its own colonial and postcolonial imprints (Prestholdt 2015), the sea's currents and flows belie similar and different spatial and historical configurations from those that mark the land. Monwabisi Resort, which was completed in 1986, forms Khayelitsha's southern border. In his research on the architecture of apartheid's segregated recreational amenities, artist Vincent Bezuidenhout (2011) noted the absence of any maps planning the building of these facilities and used contemporary aerial footage from the Department of Land Affairs to produce the composite aerial photograph *False Bay #1* (Figure 4). The image affords another reading of the configuration of "city" and "township" from the vantage point of the ocean, which takes up at least half of the frame.

Bezuidenhout portrays the Cape coastline and Strandfontein, Mnandi, Macassar, and Monwabisi, beaches designated for "Coloured" and "African" sunbathers during apartheid. As Bezuidenhout explains, the physical geography of these beaches—the ocean, dunes, and cliffs—allowed for the easy containment of people far away from the recreational facilities of the "Whites-only" Muizen-berg Beach some way up the coast. The garish design of these resorts, which resemble colonial-era British seaside pavilions, contrasts sharply with the dangerous tides and unfavorable swimming conditions for which these beaches are renowned (Bezuidenhout 2011). The design of Monwabisi—tower floodlights, controlled access through high walls, and imposing structures of concrete and face brick—mimics the appearance of Khayelitsha township and more broadly how apartheid landscaping imposed physical and psychological control. Fore-grounding the ocean is thus one way of revealing other social and historical insights that unsettle a simple positioning and narrative of Khayelitsha.

"Khayelitsha" is better thought of as a polyvalent object that is much more than its geographic location, the data that describe it in government reports and national censuses, or the varied imaginaries that circulate in research outputs, social media, and global health programs. But a close excavation of the city's colonial and apartheid history is required if we are to further understand why Cape Town and Khayelitsha are so often framed as "not the same place."

CAPE TOWN AND KHAYELITSHA: COLONIAL AND APARTHEID ORIGINS

As historian Rebekah Lee (2009, 2) observes, "Cape Town's spatial layout and still-evident racialized residential distribution attests to the city's active participa-tion in apartheid social engineering on a grand scale." The segregation of peoples by race and class in the Cape reaches back to the mid-1600s, when the Dutch established the first European settlement. The early Cape colony consisted of the Dutch settlers, indigenous Khoi and San peoples captured as slaves, and imported slaves from Dutch outposts in what is now Indonesia. Although the British abol-ished slavery in the Cape after they annexed it in 1834, they replaced it with labor regulations that perpetuated racial hierarchy (Legassick and Ross 2010). The expansion of the colony and the discovery of mineral resources in the 1870s prompted additional stringent policies to ensure a supply of cheap labor. British-Dutch tensions over sovereignty and mineral rights resulted in the Anglo-Boer War of 1899–1902 and the formation of the Union of South Africa in 1910, a British dominion. This new government ratified racial segregation laws and limited vot-ing rights to citizens designated as "White" (Freund 2011).

The 1913 Native Land Act demarcated only 7 percent of the total land of South Africa for Black ownership. As in other settler colonial contexts, such legislation led to the systematic relocation of indigenous peoples as an ongoing policy. In South Africa, Black Africans were expelled from their land to reserves through-out the twentieth century (Plaatje [1916] 1995). The National Party government that was elected in 1948 converted the reserves into ethnic bantustans in 1951 (Wylie 2001). The 1950 Population Registration Act's designation of people as either "White," "Coloured," "Indian," or "African" (Posel 2001) informed the 1950 Group Areas Act, which determined where a person could live and work based on this classification. The 1952 Natives (Abolition of Passes and Co-ordination of Documents) Act consolidated a history of requiring citizens not classified as "White" to carry a passbook that was intended to restrict people's movement. Without the required pass detailing their legitimate employment and therefore their eligibility to live closer to industrial centers, people could be charged or forcibly removed (Murray 1987). Influx control measures were particularly stringent in the Cape due to the province's Coloured Labor Preference Area Policy, which favored employees classified as "Coloured" over those classified as "African" (Goldin 1984). This policy supported the 1955 Eiselen Plan, which sought to remove all African residents from cities. In the Western Cape, those who were employed were resettled in nearby townships and those who did not have valid passes were relocated to the Transkei and Ciskei, the two rural "homelands" designated for isiXhosa speakers. These restrictions became increasingly stringent in the 1960s and 1970s as the government attempted to institute "orderly urbanization" (Murray 1987, 314). The Cape administration used an array of brutal measures, including the "repatriation" of thousands of people to the bantustans, the demolition of "illegal" settlements under the 1977 Illegal Squatting Act, and the detention of "illegals" found in the city. The early 1980s were similarly characterized by state violence in the townships of Cape Town.

The plan for Khayelitsha—a new township where the African population of Cape Town could be consolidated—was presented as a solution to the problems of overcrowding and unrest in the existing townships. The state presented this plan as a form of "community development," although local academics warned of the disastrous social and economic implications of the plan (Dewar and Watson 1984). Despite resistance from community groups, academics, and opposition parties, the construction of Khayelitsha (which means "new home" in isiXhosa) went ahead in May 1983. The initial plan consisted of three towns of four villages each in a design that facilitated internal segregation between blocks (Huchzermeyer 2003). One thousand plots of 170 square meters each were demarcated in the first phase, and tin huts and bucket toilets were allocated to each plot. Initial amenities included one school, one clinic, a mobile shop, a mobile post service, two phone booths, and a bus depot (Surplus People's Project 1984). The first residents of Khayelitsha were people who had been forced to relocate from inner-city Cape Town and residents who had moved from older townships, often to escape state-led violence in the established settlements (Dewar and Watson 1984). The apartheid regime was intent on relocating residents of the established townships of Langa, Nyanga, and Gugulethu and posed resettlement to Khayelitsha as a solution for "legal" residents of Old Crossroads and New Crossroads. In Crossroads, organized community resistance to the state's attempts to force relocations was met with a ruthless campaign of divide-and-rule tactics and state violence, culminating in 1986 in one of the most brutal forced removals in the country's history (Cole 1987). After that, Khayelitsha grew rapidly as a result of forced removals, coerced resettlement through the provision of 99-year leases for residents, and the repeal of pass laws and the Coloured Labor Preference Area Policy in 1986. The repeal of the Group Areas Act in 1991 and the accelerated urbanization that followed the democratic elections in 1994 led to further expansion.

Any account of the history of South Africa faces the difficulty of assessing the validity and verifiability of historical sources and research from the apartheid period (Lee 2009). However, a portrait of Khayelitsha in its early years can be gleaned from the urban studies, surveys, and activist documentation of events in the 1980s (Surplus People's Project 1984; Dewar and Watson 1984; Cleminshaw 1985). Anthony Mehlwana (1996) and Andrew Spiegel (Spiegel and Mehlwana 1997) conducted the first ethnography of Khayelitsha in their study of the effects of migrancy on kin networks in this settlement. Rebekah Lee's (2009) account of the lives of African women in Cape Town in the latter half of the twentieth century illustrates how second and third generations of women came to settle in Khayelitsha from townships elsewhere in the city. Khayelitsha residents thus experienced both rural-urban migrations and a series of urban relocations. Most residents retained links to rural areas and there was significant movement, or "domestic fluidity," between rural and urban areas, such that households in Khayelitsha did not conform to a nuclear pattern (Spiegel et al. 1996). Rather, Spiegel and colleagues found that "formation and reformation" of domestic arrangements in response to economic and social demands at the macro and microlevels produced a diversity of arrangements (13). The "placement and re-placement of children" occurred as resources were freed up or constrained within wider networks, or children would move between households who had forged reciprocal partnerships around child care (21; see also Reynolds 1989). Later accounts of Khayelitsha reiterate this picture of domestic flux and the con-tinuity of women at the center of these fluid social networks (du Toit et al. 2007; Skuse and Cousins 2007; Hall and Posel 2019).

KHAYELITSHA AND THE CITY

South Africa's transition to democracy, the South African Constitution, and the country's welfare programs are often cited as success stories, yet South Africa remains one of the most unequal societies in the world. Political scientists argue that the democratic transition was configured by the global turn to economic neoliberalism at the time (Bond 2007; Williams and Taylor 2010). This is reflected in the shift from policies focused on growth from redistribution and the alleviation of poverty and inequality to policies that prioritized market-led economic growth. But the account of South Africa as neoliberal overlooks the welfare protection packages that are used by one-third of the South African population. The blend of economic liberalization and social protection that characterizes contemporary South African politics might cast it more readily as a "neoliberal welfare state" (Ferguson 2015, 2). This contradiction seems especially pronounced in Cape Town, where the city has made explicit its shift in focus from the "passive government-citizen relationship" of social welfare models to a "proactive collaboration" between "the city, citizens and business" (City of Cape Town 2014).

The official narrative of Khayelitsha is as a site of investment in urban development. A massive urban renewal program has taken place there since 2001 and has produced a net increase in housing, the opening of new public spaces, new libraries, a network of clinics, a district hospital, and connections to the city's bus networks. However, this narrative does not accord with the realities of life for many Khayelitsha residents. While Cape Town's slogan until 2014 was "This City Works for You," in 2014, activist group the Tokolos Collective stenciled sidewalks, stairs, walls, doors, billboards, and road signs across the city with the message: "THIS CITY WORKS FOR A FEW."[2]

Khayelitsha is a large and diverse township that contains established sections with housing with utilities and other services, community buildings, and infrastructure; sections of heterogenous housing where brick homes built by the government stand alongside zinc dwellings; and an expanding periphery of makeshift homes without water or electricity. Modes of participation in the formal and informal economy are shaped by an individual's social capital and structural factors such as mode of transport, commuting time, and risk of exposure to crime (Du Toit and Neves 2007; Battersby 2011). Public transport is predominantly by minibus taxi. Other services, including train and bus connections, are frequently vandalized. Formal unemployment at the time of the 2011 census (the most recent at time of writing) was 38 percent. Median monthly income in that census was R2116 for men and R1526 for women, which places three-quarters of Khayelitsha households below the food poverty line.[3]

The 2011 census estimated the Khayelitsha population to be 450,000 residents, but some argue that the figure may have been closer to one million (Brunn and Wilson 2013). In that census, 98.7 percent of residents describe themselves as Black African. The most commonly spoken language is isiXhosa, followed by English. Age groups 20–24 and 25–29 represent larger cohorts in the census than other age groups because of the high rate of migration of young adults to Khayelitsha (Statistics South Africa 2013).

Since 1994, development efforts have failed to keep up with continued population expansion, and a sprawl of informal settlements that make up around 50 percent of the township now surrounds the original area designated for Khayelitsha. According to census data, at least half of Khayelitsha's population lives in informal dwellings. Other sources suggest that at least 10,000 new informal homes are erected in Khayelitsha every year (Affordable Land & Housing Data Centre 2013). Sixty percent of residents have access to piped water, sixty percent have electricity, seventy percent have access to a flush toilet, and eighty-five percent have their refuse removed weekly. Thousands of residents who live outside these serviced areas rely on shared taps and a dysfunctional bucket toilet system.

In contrast, consider the suburb of Claremont, a historically privileged part of the city of similar geographical size, about 35 square kilometers, that was designated "Whites-only" in 1969. The population of Claremont in 2011 was 17,198 residents. Sixty-four percent of the population identified as "White," 95 percent described themselves as employed, 77 percent earned more than R6,400 per month,[4] and 99.5 percent were living in formal housing with access to piped water, flush toilets, and electricity. The stark inequalities in income and life circumstances for Capetonians are reflected in South Africa's Gini coefficient;[5] it is the highest in the world (World Bank 2019).

The census data for Khayelitsha reflect the circumstances of the women in the present study. The study cohort also accords with the migration patterns and living arrangements of Khayelitsha residents described in previous work.

CHARACTERISTICS OF THE STUDY COHORT

In this group of fifteen participants, Nobomi, age 21, was the youngest, and Songezwa, age 33, was the oldest. Two-thirds of the group were from the Eastern Cape province and had moved to Khayelitsha in early childhood, for high school, or for work after completing schooling. Nonyameko had come specifically for the birth of her child. Of the five women born in the Western Cape, Nobomi, Lindiwe, and Nocawe had all been born in Khayelitsha and Bathandwa and Fezeka had been born in nearby townships and had moved to Khayelitsha later in childhood. Two-thirds of the women were unemployed. Of those that worked, only Inam had work requiring a college degree and worked in the media. Lindiwe and Veliswa had both obtained university diplomas; Lindiwe worked in a factory and Veliswa worked as a teacher. Aviwe, Nocawe, and Nonyameko had jobs as domestic workers. Aviwe and Nocawe had completed a few years of secondary school, and Nonyameko had only completed primary school. Khanyiswa was the only one who was currently pursuing post-secondary education; she was taking classes at a local technical college. Of those who were not employed, Bathandwa, Fezeka, and Ndileka had completed secondary school, while Lumka, Nobomi, Anele, Nandipha, and Songezwa had stopped short of finishing their schooling. All of the women sought state child support grants (320 rand or thirty US dollars at that time) except for Inam and Veliswa, who both earned more than the income threshold for eligibility.

The women's living arrangements reflect the diversity of household composition in Khayelitsha. Some households resembled the nuclear family model:

Aviwe, Nocawe, Ndileka, Lumka, Songezwa, Bathandwa, and Veliswa lived with their husbands and children. Nandipha was the only one living alone with her partner before the birth of their first child. Khanyiswa lived with her sister in a house that belonged to their father; Anele lived with her cousin. Nonyameko lived with two friends. Others lived in extended households. Inam lived with her mother, her sister, her nieces, a cousin, and her first child. Lindiwe also lived with her mother, her cousin, and her first child while Fezeka and Nobomi lived in extended households with mothers, aunts, siblings, or cousins.

Housing and household amenities also varied among the participants. Bathandwa, Veliswa, Inam, Lindiwe, Khanyiswa, Nandipha, Fezeka and Nobomi lived in brick houses with electricity and running water. Bathandwa and her husband were the only participants who owned several properties in Khayelitsha that they rented out for additional income. Aviwe, Nocawe, Ndileka, Anele, Nonyameko, Songezwa and Lumka lived in zinc dwellings that were electrified, but they depended on shared taps and shared toilets for water and sanitation. The size and condition of zinc homes varied considerably. Aviwe lived in a large zinc home with multiple rooms, including a kitchen equipped with stove and a washing machine, while Nonyameko, Ndileka, Songezwa, and Anele lived in single-room shacks. If we arrived at Ndileka's house in the morning, we would find her packing away the rat traps from the previous evening—illegal poisons that many Khayelitsha residents use to manage the persistent problem of rodent infestation (Levine et al. 2020). None of the households had a water heater and hot water was obtained by boiling a kettle. All the households had televisions, and the women who lived in brick housing tended to subscribe to paid television services. Nandipha was the only participant who had a personal computer at home.

For the majority of the women in this study, life was characterized by significant movement between Khayelitsha and homes located predominantly in the Eastern Cape, especially over the December holiday period (see Figure 5). But it is wise to avoid any overdetermination of what "rural" means in relation to Khayelitsha. As Zolani Ngwane (2003) shows in his analysis of "Christmas time" in the Eastern Cape, circulations between these homes do not fit into a dominant model of urbanization, and Rebekah Lee (2009) has documented how perceptions and experiences of the so-called rural-urban divide differ across generations. Khayelitsha's position on the rural-urban axis is thus another set of coordinates that decenters common configurations of township, city, and homestead.

SITUATED BIOLOGIES

Khayelitsha's disease burden is often cited as emblematic of South Africa's "four concurrent epidemics": HIV/AIDS, infectious diseases and undernutrition, noncommunicable diseases, and trauma related to high rates of violence and bodily injury (Coovadia et al. 2009, 817). The township has close to the highest

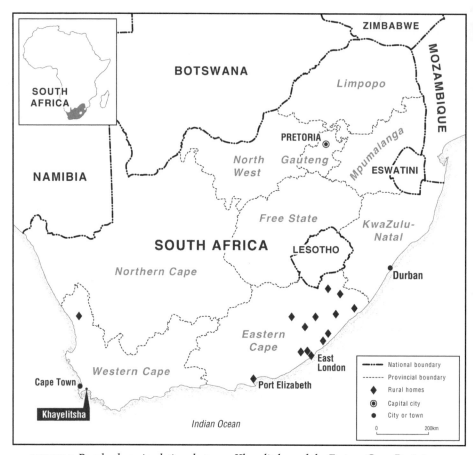

FIGURE 5. Rural-urban circulations between Khayelitsha and the Eastern Cape. Participants left Khayelitsha periodically for their other homes (represented by diamonds), which were predominantly located in the Eastern Cape. (Map by Miles Irving)

rates of HIV and tuberculosis infection in the world. One in three women test positive for HIV when they enroll for antenatal health care and tuberculosis is endemic; the incidence is at least 1,500 per 100,000 cases per year (Médecins Sans Frontières 2011). High rates of child undernutrition have been documented in the area since the 1980s (Le Roux and Le Roux 1991), while the prevalence of obesity is higher than the national average (Malhotra et al. 2008). This is associated with a substantial burden of noncommunicable diseases (Puoane et al. 2012). In addition, the Khayelitsha Commission (2014, 44) showed that Khayelitsha "has the highest numbers of murders, attempted murders, sexual offences, assault with intent to do grievous bodily harm and robbery with aggravating circumstances nationwide."

Khayelitsha's complex health profile originates in the specific intersections of its physical landscape and climate, its political history, its social geography, its built environment, and the globalized economy (Pentecost and Cousins 2017). In lieu of interpretations of epigenetic science that might understand "the environment" as an object that can be well circumscribed, anthropologists Jorg Niewöhner and Margaret Lock (2018, 692) use the term "situated biologies" to "point to the ubiquity of the co-constitutional processes of matter and meaning and of human and environment."

Geomorphology, climate, energy usage, high-density living in rudimentary housing, and sociopolitical and economic exclusion all contribute to a syndemic of HIV, tuberculosis, other infectious diseases, malnutrition, and noncommunicable diseases in Khayelitsha.[6] High rates of respiratory illness reflect both cramped living conditions and the area's topography. Khayelitsha lies in the Southern Cape Condensation Problem Area, an area between East London and Malmesbury that has higher rates of condensation due to a combination of higher rainfall and wind patterns created by the Southern Cape mountain ranges. This phenomenon causes a higher risk of respiratory disease for residents of the Condensation Problem Area (Matthews et al. 2003). Khayelitsha's air quality is also the worst in Cape Town; pollutants measure seventy times higher there than in the central business district, compounded by dust from the dunes and the burning of waste, wood, and rubber in the township (Muchapondwa 2010). Inadequacies in sanitation and water contamination in the area also affects the health of both people and livestock, manifesting in diarrheal disease that results in increased risk of child malnutrition and mortality (Social Justice Coalition and Ndifuna Ukwazi 2014).

Against the backdrop of this nutrition-sanitation nexus is a dual burden of child undernutrition and adult obesity in Khayelitsha that reflects a national trend. Since the mid-1990s, South Africa's food system has been characterized by the expansion of supermarket chains, intensified food marketing practices, increased foreign direct investment in food production and distribution, and incorporation into global markets. Foreign investment since 1994 has aided the consolidation of power by corporations that include the national enterprises Tiger Brands and Pioneer Foods and transnational giants Nestlé, Unilever, Parmalat, Danone, Kraft, and PepsiCo—so-called Big Food (Igumbor et al. 2012). Supermarket chains, which have expanded rapidly in South Africa since 1994, dominate both urban and rural sectors. While these chains provide staples and packaged foods at a lower cost to the population, the healthier foods they sell are consistently more expensive than nutrient-poor alternatives (Temple and Steyn 2009). Like the majority of South Africans, Khayelitsha residents consume a diet of low dietary diversity.

As is the case in other townships in South Africa, most food in Khayelitsha is supplied by one of a handful of supermarket conglomerates. Street vendors,

TABLE 1   Price comparison between different food outlets in Khayelitsha
in 2015

	Price Chain	Shoprite	Spaza shop
10 kg maize meal	R69.99	R69.99	R70
10 kg rice	R110	R112.49	R105
10 kg flour	R89.99	R85.99	R85
10 kg sugar	R99.99	R84.99	R110
2 litres cooking oil	R31.99	R32.95	R35
2.5 kg samp	R19.99	R19.99	R25
500 g beans	R14.99	R15	R18
2 litres milk	R17.99	R19.99	R18
1 loaf white bread	R9.99	R10.49	R11
1 loaf brown bread	R8.99	R8.99	R10
2 kg braai meat	R42.99	R44.99	R45
155 g tinned fish	R7.99	R7.99	R9
750 g corn flake cereal	R35.99	R39.99	Not available
175 g soap	R8.99	R8.99	R10
1 kg washing powder	R30.99	R32.99	R33

spaza shops (informal convenience shops), and shebeens (drinking taverns) also dot Khayelitsha's landscape. Spazas, which are in walking distance for most residents, sell basic provisions through small, grated windows to protect owners from theft. Spazas stock staples including bread, tinned beans, maize meal and processed food such as chips, soft drinks, and sweets. Vendors and roadside food stalls sell chips and muffins, amagwinya (fried dough), shisinyama (grilled meat), Russians (smoked sausages), and smileys (grilled sheep heads). Corporations such as Coca-Cola and Nestlé access this economy using "bottom of the pyramid" entrepreneurship models that deliver their commodities through "micro-entrepreneurs" (Dolan 2012, 4) and increase their brand presence by supplying free refrigeration, bicycles, displays, and uniforms (Nestlé South Africa 2013), in addition to ubiquitous signage on every street corner ("Coke and Meals Go Better Together"). Table 1 compares the prices of basic commodities at a bulk-buy outlet (Price Chain), a supermarket (Shoprite), and a spaza shop in Khayelitsha during the time of the study. In accordance with a 2020 study (Odunitan-Wayas 2021), my observation was that fruit and vegetables were less available and often of poorer quality in Khayelitsha's food outlets than in more affluent parts of Cape Town.

The noncommunicable diseases burden in Khayelitsha reflects both the built environment and sociopolitical and economic factors (Smit et al. 2015). Rates of malnutrition and associated metabolic diseases and mental health disorders are influenced by chronic food insecurity, lack of opportunity for safe physical activity, and high rates of stress and depression (Smit et al. 2015). A 2011 study documented chronic food insecurity in 89 percent of Khayelitsha households in a seasonal pattern that has two troughs: in January, likely due to less employment and greater demands on existing resources during the festive season, and in June, likely as a result of fewer labor opportunities during inclement winter weather (Battersby 2011).[7] Food insecurity has a strong association with postnatal depression, hazardous drinking, and suicidal ideation in women in Khayelitsha (Dewing et al. 2013). Physical activity is constrained by a lack of safe public spaces for exercise, while high rates of crime also exacerbate stress and anxiety (Smit et al. 2015).

The next chapter shows how, despite these complexities, policies consistently circumscribe "the environment" to the maternal body and the nuclear family, enjoining pregnant women to consume a healthy diet, exercise regularly, prepare for breastfeeding, and engage as an active liberal subject responsible for intergenerational health outcomes. Such a framing falls apart in spectacular fashion against the very real constraints of life configured by racialized spatial regimes of violence that have relegated people to inhospitable environs.

3 · THE TRAVELING TECHNOLOGY OF MOTHER AND CHILD

"Combating the transgenerational risk of noncommunicable diseases in transitioning societies." This was the theme of the ninth World Congress on Developmental Origins of Health and Disease, held in Cape Town in November 2015. Emblazoned on conference banners and posters at the Cape Town International Convention Centre, these words encapsulated the DOHaD field's concerns with the transgenerational transmission of noncommunicable diseases, particularly in so-called transitioning societies. An eminent South African scientist who introduced the proceedings highlighted the statement that nowhere was this research more relevant than in the local context. "In terms of Africa and in particular South Africa, we are experiencing transition in a very rapid time," he stated. The scientist outlined the complexity of the South African situation, which included the concurrent epidemics of obesity and HIV and the lack of knowledge about the potential epigenetic effects of antiretroviral treatment during pregnancy. He concluded by affirming the particular importance of DOHaD research in this and similar contexts.

I was seated in the audience in the plush conference hall, which was laid out like a cinema theater with burgundy curtains and red velvet seats. Two huge banners reading "DOHaD 2015" flanked the stage. A British scientist gave the next presentation, which outlined the emergence of the field, or "the developmental origins of DOHaD," as the speaker quipped. He paid homage to David Barker as the founding father of DOHaD and traced the evolution of the field from the inaugural conference in Mumbai in 1990. He ended with a PowerPoint slide featuring the DOHaD logo: a fetus nestled in a womb in the shape of the earth. After noting its similarity to a breech presentation, he made the somewhat provocative joke that as usual, "the brain and the placenta are in the North, and the South can take care of the nether regions." Africa, he suggested, is "the omphalos"—the source of nourishment. The global imaginary evoked here—of the belly of Africa as the primordial womb—has long authorized intervention on the continent (Bayart 1993), most notably for the figure of the mother and child (Vaughan 1991).

I attended the three-day conference as a presenter on one of the poster panels. That this conference took place in Cape Town was not just serendipitous for my fieldwork but also a confirmation of the strong presence of DOHaD research in South African science. The DOHaD focus on the Global South was evident in the range of large-scale studies presented, which were being conducted in the Gambia, South Africa, Tanzania, Chile, Brazil, India, and the West Indies. As the symposium's theme stated, these "transitioning societies" are the core target of DOHaD interventions. I was attending both as a clinician with special interests in perinatology and the epidemiology of metabolic diseases and as an anthropologist of science and policy. I presented initial ethnographic findings on the disjunctures between the food environments of urban township residents in Cape Town and South African perinatal nutrition policy, which by 2015 was directly informed by DOHaD discourses.

In this chapter, I examine how discourse travels, how it comes to shape health care delivery on the ground, and the modes of governance and self-governance it legitimizes. The chapter is divided into three parts, each of which addresses an important element in the first 1,000 days discourse. The ethnography moves from sites of policy and knowledge production to the clinic as a mediating site of ideas and then to domestic spaces as a site for intervention. I have organized the material in this way to provide a detailed illustration of how global discourses of health shape interventions and how these interventions come to bear on everyday life in Khayelitsha. As mentioned in the introduction, Khayelitsha is a research archipelago (Rottenburg 2009) where the focus on the first 1,000 days is only of many policies aimed at maternal and child health and one of many public health and research regimes and interventions. My key argument in this chapter is that these interventions share an ideological figuration of "the maternal" and "the child" (see also Castañeda 2002) that permits certain forms of paternalistic governance in a specified population: mothers and infants. In this chapter I evidence the first tenet of what I describe as a politics of potential: the substance of potential is perceived as located in particular subjects and not in others. I trace this argument from policy that targets the economic potential of early life interventions through to the particularities of maternal roles in what James Ferguson (2015, 9) terms the "African social."

DOHAD AND NONCOMMUNICABLE DISEASES: SHIFTING CATEGORIES OF DISEASE IN SOUTH AFRICA'S POLICY DISCOURSE

The 2015 DOHaD congress showcased the first 1,000 days approach as a cost-effective project to decrease the transgenerational risk of noncommunicable

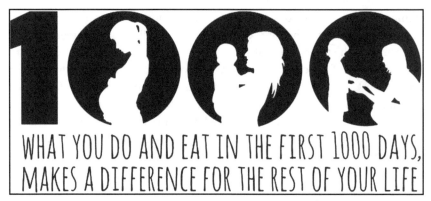

FIGURE 6. Poster on display at the 2015 DOHaD World Congress. (Photographed by the author, November 2015. © Nutricia)

diseases. The conference devoted an entire panel to "life course economics," which included presentations on "Childhood Exposures and Adult Human Capital" and the "Best Buys in the First 1,000 Days for South Africa." There was also a strong corporate presence at the conference. Representatives from Nestlé, Danone, and Novo Nordisk presented on topics such as "Public-Private Partnerships in NCD [Noncommunicable Diseases] Prevention," and during lunch breaks delegates were invited to explore interactive first 1,000 days displays (Figure 6). A key message of the conference was that evidence that has an economic rationale is more easily translated into policy and that DOHaD science needed to focus on methodologies that could address this, such as better longitudinal cohort data analysis and how to conduct robust preconception studies. I heard this fiscal argument for the first 1,000 days focus throughout my interactions with academics, public health officials, and policymakers.

The perceived cost effectiveness of early life interventions and the currency of the mother-child dyad in the humanitarian imagination have revived interest in and funding for maternal and child health interventions. As one public health specialist summarized it for me: "As soon as you say we're going to focus on pregnant women and children, then you get somewhere." Researchers and practitioners frequently referred to the fiscal logic of early life interventions using the language of "investments and returns," "maximizing chances," "scaling up," and getting "bang for your buck."[1] In a funding climate that privileges instrumental and targeted approaches, it is not surprising that researchers and advocates cite the return of "$3 for every $1 invested" (Fink et al. 2016, 104) as an incentive for investment in this area. The economic logic of the first 1,000 days is about using capital efficiently in the present and creating healthy (profit-making) human capital in the future. It is a prime example of what Michelle Murphy (2017) has termed "the economization of life"—the financialization of the rela-

tions between life, reproduction, and capital such that life itself may be categorized as either life worthy of investment or life that will offer diminishing
economic returns. The appeal of the first 1,000 days rests on the tantalizing economic promise that it will both produce an economically productive work force
and lower the health care bill for future generations. As one epidemiologist put
it, optimal early life nutrition will not only have immediate benefits but will also
alleviate the growing burden of noncommunicable diseases.

In South Africa, noncommunicable diseases are one of the elements of the
country's "quadruple burden of disease." In a seminar delivered at Stellenbosch
University in late 2014, the chief director of Metro District Health in the Western
Cape outlined four disease categories of focus for the province's Healthcare 2030
Road to Wellness plan: (1) HIV and tuberculosis, (2) trauma, (3) noncommunicable diseases, and (4) "communicable, maternal, perinatal and nutritional conditions" (Western Cape Department of Health 2014). He described South Africa
as having "developing-country syndrome" and cited Khayelitsha as a key example, where "all four are causes of death." Throughout my fieldwork, it was not
uncommon for Khayelitsha to be presented as the most fitting illustration of the
country's key syndemics. The description of a "quadruple burden" for public
health, however, has evolved over time. "Chronic diseases of lifestyle"—obesity,
cardiovascular disease, diabetes mellitus, hypertension (Steyn et al. 2006)—now
fall within the category of "noncommunicable diseases." "Infectious" diseases are
now framed as "communicable." "Communicable, maternal, perinatal, and nutritional conditions" are now considered to be part of a discrete category. While the
implicit link between infection, nutrition, and maternal and child health is not
new, the inclusion of new kinds of communicability in the framing of a certain
nexus of pathology is new in this formulation. In DOHaD frameworks, early life
nutrition now predicts a potential future risk of noncommunicable diseases;
older notions of communicability are now expanded to include what was previously labeled as noncommunicable.

I discussed the Healthcare 2030 Road to Wellness framework with a researcher
on the Western Cape Department of Health's epidemiological surveillance team
a few weeks after the chief director's presentation. She referred to the 2011 Western Cape Mortality Profile (Groenewald et al. 2014), which used the classification the chief director had referred to in order to categorize causes of mortality
in the Western Cape province into four "broad cause" groups: Group I, HIV/
AIDS and tuberculosis; Other Group I, communicable, maternal, perinatal, and
nutritional diseases; Group II, noncommunicable diseases; and Group III, injuries. The creation of a provincial mortality profile using cause of death data is a
useful exercise for presenting a picture of the province's most pressing health
issues, and it informs funding allocations. However, what constitutes nutritional
causes of mortality in this picture is not clear. "Nutritional conditions" are ill
defined in the Western Cape Mortality Profile (Groenewald et al. 2014) and in

the Healthcare 2030 Road to Wellness framework (Western Cape Department of Health 2014). The epidemiologist explained that the reason nutrition was grouped with communicable diseases and maternal and child health was that together these constituted "diseases of poverty". The reasoning behind this grouping of mortality rates may reflect the new scientific evidence that links these conditions, but it might also reflect implicit judgments. The underlying assumption is that women and children are most afflicted by diseases of poverty, a reflection of long-standing views in public health about vulnerability (Wheeler 1985; Zarowsky et al. 2013).

Ultimately the new "quadruple burden" articulated in the report and the provincial government's 2030 plan reflects changing categories of disease importance informed by the wider shift to a focus on noncommunicable diseases, the (re)emergence of maternal and child health as a prominent focus of health policy, and the implicit linkage of the perinatal period with conditions associated with nutrition. In sum, as frameworks incorporate new science, policy categories and targets are recalibrated with clear outcomes for resource allocation.

The national reconfiguration of policy priorities filters down to influence health care delivery in the province through provincial policy directives, new protocols, revised allocations of funding, and staff training. I had a better sense of the actualities of this process after interviewing an official at the Western Cape Department of Health. The department's offices in central Cape Town are located in a marble-floored building that has a well-dressed concierge. Its façade is deceiving, though; inside, it is a maze of open-plan partitioned desks covered in stacks of paper. My interviewee's office was packed with piles of documents, cardboard boxes, office supplies, pamphlets, flip files, and clipboards. On his door was a long-defunct sign that said Countdown to MDGs: ____ Days.

He explained that national policy, which involves all of the district stakeholders who are involved in implementation, informs the development of protocols in South Africa's nine provinces. In the Western Cape, both the nutrition directorate and the women's health directorate were involved in the formulation of the new basic antenatal care protocols because the new nutrition policy was largely directed at the antenatal and early postnatal periods. "The women's health, nutrition and child health subdirectorates now sit together around this issue," the official explained. "At our annual review meeting, the emphases were on maternal and child health and on noncommunicable diseases. A great emphasis was placed on getting it right in the first 1,000 days, because if we can get the infant off on the right start, we can prepare him for a healthy lifestyle later. . . . The new policy places a lot of emphasis on the importance of maternal nutrition." He underlined the role in the new protocol of intensive counseling for all women. "We felt that with a normal pregnancy, you know, when a woman is of normal weight, she also needs counseling about maintaining her weight. . . . We feel that obesity is where we should be focusing." The implications of the health official's words—that intensifying the focus on obesity requires closer attention to maternal nutrition—reflects a belief that mothers are responsible for obesity rates that has been well documented elsewhere (Maher et al. 2010; McNaughton 2011; Warin et al. 2012).

The first 1,000 days idea was also shaping policy in other areas of government, notably the Department of Education. Speaking at a workshop in Stellenbosch titled "Overcoming Poverty and Inequality" in 2014, the superintendent general of the Western Cape Department of Education presented the new 2015 "0–4 years" curriculum. The superintendent spent considerable time on the role of mothers in this early life period and made her argument in economic terms. "There are things you can do to improve childhood development that cost no money," she explained, "like educating the mothers." She made a clear link between maternal education and the capacity to parent effectively: "Just keep getting the girls to Matric because they are more likely to look after their children if they are educated."[2]

The words of the health official and the superintendent reveal a paternalistic logic rooted in a gendered and individualized sense of maternal responsibility that traverses the health and education sectors. Following the long-standing focus in international development on young girls, interventions for nutrition and early childhood development target young mothers, and increasingly all women capable of conception (Pentecost and Meloni 2020).

The renewed interest in the maternal body as a key site of intervention in global health policy is thus constituted by a shift to a focus on noncommunicable diseases, a simultaneous formalization of DOHaD and epigenetics as research fields, and a widening focus to include the preconception period. This collective global knowledge now shapes national and provincial nutrition policy in South Africa, and the key implementation site for that policy is the clinic.

THE CLINIC AS MEDIATING SITE

I had been conducting fieldwork for a few months in two of Khayelitsha's clinics when a stack of new booklets on the first 1,000 days appeared in the Sunrise Clinic's observation room, where pregnant women have their weight and blood pressure recorded. The nurse in charge told me that they would be dispensed to every pregnant woman attending the clinic. The pocket-sized, peach-colored booklet unfolded into a large poster. The brochure's title, *Feeding Smart from the Start,* was accompanied by a stylized image of a Black African woman feeding an infant. It explained:

> The first 1000 days of a child's life (from when a woman falls pregnant to when her child turns 2) is a very important time for shaping a child's ability to grow and

develop. Pregnant moms should eat a variety of healthy foods that are rich in vitamins and minerals. When moms eat well, so do their babies.

These messages are brought to you by the South African Department of Health: Nutrition Directorate and GAIN (Global Alliance for Improved Nutrition).

In addition to the clinic's official information for mothers on the importance of the early life period, NGOs also displayed posters in the clinic. A poster in the waiting room conveyed this message:

> Molweni bomama! [Hello mothers!] We would like to talk to you about your babies. . . . We are taking the first 3 years of life very seriously because it is during this time that the foundation is laid down for the future development of the child. . . . If you are feeling well then your baby will feel well and develop in the way you want it to. Just as you pay attention to your baby's physical needs, like food and immunization, so you must pay attention to your own and your baby's emotional needs.

The pamphlets and posters all feature the mother-child dyad as an explicit visual location of the desired intervention, which in this case is the exhortation of pregnant women and mothers to eat a variety of healthy foods and attend to their emotional well-being to ensure a healthy foundation for "the future development of the child." These materials thus convey the politics of potential: where it is to be found (the dyad), who might be responsible for manifesting it (pregnant women and mothers), and when the fruits of that work might appear (in the future). While the poster's focus on the effects of maternal mental health is relatively new, the pamphlet's focus on "eating well" in pregnancy follows a long line of interventions that have targeted maternal nutrition, of which the clinic is a material catalog.

The Clinic as Catalog

The clinic can be considered a kind of catalog of the various international strategies directed toward malnutrition. It is a catalog in the archival sense (Foucault 1972) that the clinic's materiality—infrastructure, posters, leaflets and protocols— evidence older interventions, and in the dynamic sense, given that clinical practice is unevenly informed by interventions and campaigns that have historically shaped care, such as the selective primary health care strategies of the 1980s and the focus on micronutrients in later interventions. The first 1,000 days—a new formulation of a long-standing focus on the perinatal period—thus travels alongside older frameworks for perinatal care, reflected in the everyday interactions of clinic staff and the materiality of the space where they conduct their work.

That maternal and child health and nutrition has long been a primary health care focus in the two clinics of this study was evident in the visual catalog of health care campaigns on the clinic's walls. In the reception area of one clinic, a large mural depicts the stages of a child's first five years of life—a baby on all fours, a standing toddler, and finally a small child playing with colorful blocks. A rudimentary clinic card is painted in the top right-hand corner with a list: "birth, 6 weeks, 10 weeks, 14 weeks, 9 months, 18 months, 5 years," with the isiXhosa message: "Abantwana bam basempilweni kuba ndibagonyisile ukuya kwimin-yaka emihlanu" (All of my children are healthy, because they received all of their immunizations until five years). The mural was painted by local medical students after the clinic opened in 2005. Other familiar public health messages appear in posters around the clinic:

"Your child needs vitamin A. Take your child to the clinic every 6 months until the age of 5 years."

"Introduce solids from 6 months. Fruit and vegetables are important."

"Exclusive breastfeeding for 6 months is the best nutrition for your baby."

"Adequate nutrition during infancy and early childhood is important in the development of each child's potential."

The clinic's paraphernalia thus illustrated the continuities of new policy with pre-existing perinatal protocols. What set the first 1,000 days policy apart from some of its predecessors was the explicit link it made to adult health outcomes for the infant subjects of the intervention. The changing visual material landscape of the clinic might thus be viewed as a dynamic catalog of interventions in early life.

The catalog was also evident in the language and comportment of clinic staff, and in their techniques and practices of clinical care. In a clinical education session for nursing students that I observed, the stern, elderly nursing sister overseeing the session employed the GOBI-FFF acronym (growth, oral rehy-dration, breastfeeding, immunization, food supplementation, female literacy, family planning) to direct her clinical practice and teaching, rather than the newer framework officially used at the clinic, the Integrated Management of Childhood Illness, which was endorsed by the National Department of Health and the World Health Organization. "Now we're going to do the GOBI-FFF," she said to the nursing students, one of whom was tasked with conducting the consultation with a mother and her six-week-old infant who had been recruited from the queue for this practical teaching session. Starting with "growth," the nursing students noted that the baby was growing well according to the growth chart. "As long as your baby grows all along the line it is good," the senior nurse explained to the mother. "Just make sure that the weight goes along the green line. If it goes above the line, it indicates overweight. If under the line, under-weight. Good. Now we will talk about oral rehydration. What do you know about it?" The mother knew that it was a mixture of some kind but was unsure what it consisted of, so the nurse explained that, should the infant have diarrhea, the mother should make up a rehydration solution using 1 liter of cooled boiled water, six teaspoons of sugar, and half a teaspoon of salt. Moving on to breast-feeding, the nurse asked the mother when she feeds the baby. "When he makes that sound," the mother responded. She mimicked the infant's grimace to explain, and this satisfied the nurse. "Good! She is demand feeding. You should change nappies six to eight times per day, mama, that is normal. You should breastfeed only until six months then add vegetables. You should also play and talk and sing to the baby to stimulate it. Have you applied for a child grant for the baby yet?" "Not yet." "Are you using family planning?"

This infant's immunizations were up to date according to his Road to Health booklet. This booklet is distributed to South African parents following an infant's birth and is supposed to be used at clinic visits to track a wide range of health data.[3] As Lenore Manderson and Fiona Ross (2005) have noted, the Road to Health Booklet makes "no record of maternal or social well-being" (5). There is therefore no prompt for queries about this, and at no point in the conversation did the nurse inquire about the mother's health, except to note that she should get her blood pressure checked again. No inquiry was made about the child's father or other caregivers.

The senior nurse ticked off the GOBI-FFF items, sticking to close-ended questions that quickly satisfied the protocol. In place of asking how the mother was doing or allowing her to express any concerns, the questions were carefully framed to ensure that the consultation was performed efficiently. When the nursing sister asked if the mother had applied for a child support grant yet—the closest she came to inquiring about the mother's present social situation—the answer "not yet" was quickly passed over and there was no follow-up about whether the mother knew how to apply for this grant. This interaction could be construed as a small example of the "selective primary care" GOBI-FFF promoted, a more feasible and cost-effective option than the comprehensive "health care for all" that was the initial goal of primary health care set out in the 1978 Alma Ata Declaration. What is most noteworthy about it is the nurse's continued use of the acronym as a teaching tool, which shows how older or outdated discourses of maternal and child health continue to circulate in the clinic and how they continue to privilege infant health over women's health in the postpartum period.

The younger nurses I interviewed were all familiar with the newer protocol, the Integrated Management of Childhood Illness endorsed by the World Health Organization. One staff member explained this as important because the protocol also included looking for danger signs such as swollen feet, a protruding stomach, or a skin condition. "The baby might have a normal weight and the mid-upper arm circumference might be normal, but you need to check these signs," he explained. The language used to describe conditions of undernutrition also differed—some staff members continued to use the language of "kwashiorkor" and "marasmus" to describe what others referred to as "protein-energy malnutrition with or without edema."

The protocols and terminologies staff used likely reflect those that were in use at the time of their training. However, nursing staff were scheduled to attend additional training and professional development sessions held by the health directorate once or twice a year on a rotating roster; therefore, some staff were more familiar with newer clinical protocols than others. In the case of the new nutrition policy, the health promotions officer and the nurses responsible for antenatal and infant care had attended workshops first and communicated these ideas in the weekly breastfeeding support group meetings.

Communicating Notions of Transgenerational Disease

Sr. Qoma[4] held breastfeeding support sessions on Friday afternoons in her consulting room. On one particular day, four women attended and it was a tight squeeze to get the mothers, their infants, their baby bags and blankets, Sr. Qoma, me, and my research assistant into the small office. One of the young women sat on the examination bed, two sat on plastic chairs, and one was offered Sr. Qoma's swiveling desk chair. Nomsa and I stood against a small counter behind the desk and Sr. Qoma stood at her desk for the duration of the session. She started by delivering information about infant weight and breastfeeding, illustrating with the Road to Health booklet. "The weight should be between these lines," she said, pointing to the centiles on the chart. She explained that if the baby falls below the line, he is underweight and if he is above the line, overweight. She went through each page in the health booklet, from basic information to vaccination schedules, speaking rapidly. "You should breastfeed exclusively whether you are HIV positive or negative. You breastfeed your baby for six months. You don't give the baby water or anything else—you just breastfeed. If you mix feed there is a possibility that the child will be sick when he is older; he may get a disease."

During this initial advice, the clinic's health promotions officer, Ms. Tyani, arrived and leaned against the door of the crowded room. She interjected:

When you mix feed your child, that inwebu [lining] can disappear [referring to the gut]. So whatever you give the child, it goes in that gut and it makes cracks, and those cracks are the entry point to any virus. That can happen to a child whether they are HIV positive or HIV negative. So you can't give a child food at all, at all. If you mix feed, you are introducing the baby to diabetes, to hypertension. Your child can get diabetes or hypertension because you as a parent, you introduced her to food at an early age. Those chemicals, they increase the pressure of a child to get fat, and then you will always have to go to the clinic. . . . I'm sorry I'm late, I just wanted to add this thing. . . . I just so wish that you would all continue breastfeeding. Start bit by bit. A journey of 1,000 miles starts with only one step. Only one step!

Ms. Tyani's animated delivery did little to rouse the group, who were somewhat less interactive than what the term "support group" might suggest. Sr. Qoma delivered a barrage of information and then the health promotions officer did the same. Both Sr. Qoma and Ms. Tyani took pains to impress on the young women the very serious consequences of not breastfeeding exclusively for six months regardless of HIV status and made an explicit link between "mixed feeding" and the possibility of disease later in life, based on an understanding that the infant gut is vulnerable and that "chemicals" in food can enter the gut and have long-lasting effects on health. A clear message was given that feeding practices in early infancy can affect the risk of overweight, diabetes, and hypertension. The session was thus a moment when the clinic served as a mediating site between the new nutrition policy and the clinic "clients," as staff members referred to them.

The women I observed in the clinic were frequently passive in the face of the often-brusque, efficient, and prescriptive instructions the nursing staff meted out, but they occasionally challenged advice or sought clarification. As the senior nurse educator had, both Sr. Qoma and Ms. Tyani asked the mothers close-ended questions, such as "Has the baby had immunizations yet?" and "Are you breast-feeding exclusively?" One young woman responded that her husband wanted the child to have both breast milk and formula to assist with weight gain. "We are always fighting, my husband and I, because he wants me to give the baby formula. We are always arguing about this thing. So it is not easy for me. . . . Every time the baby cries, he wants to give the baby formula. I tried to explain to him that things are different now, there are other diseases now, so it is a risk to give the baby for-mula." The health promotions officer responded by impressing on the woman the need to "explain" to her husband. "Basically, you need to make him understand," she offered. As on many other occasions, male partners' concerns were dismissed. Another young mother asked about what she should do when she returned to work, and both the nurse and health promoter discussed expressing breast milk and using a peanut butter jar to store milk, ensuring that containers are sterile and that the milk would be warmed by the person feeding the baby. They did not ask whether this would be practical for the woman's particular situation.

After the support group, I interviewed Ms. Tyani to clarify some of the advice we had heard her give the young mothers: "This idea that whatever we eat deter-mines if we get chronic disease—you were talking about that in relation to what you introduce at an early age. Could you expand on that for me?" Ms. Tyani gave a detailed response:

Do they know how big their children's stomachs are? Because you find that it is challenging for this stomach, because of the amount of food that you . . . because the stomach it is a muscle . . . the amount of food that you put in that stomach, it is going to accommodate because it stretches, so the child is going to grow know-ing larger amounts of food in her stomach, you understand? So the child is not developing the right way the child is supposed to be developing. He or she is going to be overweight; she is going to understand *the language* of being overweight, you understand? So when the child is overweight, he or she is at stake [risk] of getting this hypertension, this diabetes, those chest problems, because now her lungs are so squeezed up with fat and whatever, it is difficult for the child to breathe, you understand, because those chronic diseases, they don't start when the child is old, you introduce your child at an early age, you know, just mixed feeding him, or giving all that food, all those proteins, unnecessary protein, all the fat that a child is not supposed to be getting.

Ms. Tyani explained that she had attended a recent workshop run by the Department of Health where they had explained these concepts. "It included the stuff that we are normally trained on, but this was one was a bit advanced," she said. One of the nurses had also learned these concepts at a recent training session. "What I've learnt about is the problems with the gut, that babies have ulcers in later life that may even lead to cancer. Especially with the HIV-positive mothers. Today if someone has a problem with ulcers in the stomach and they don't know why, maybe it is because they were fed early," she explained. It is unclear where staff received these incorrect ideas. During fieldwork in the clinic from August to December 2014, the precepts of the new nutrition policy were implemented in a stepwise fashion, with staff being trained one by one and new posters and pamphlets arriving in stages. What interested me most was how patients understood the new notions of intergenerational health and disease that these communicated.

Theory from the Waiting Room

The words of new parents in the waiting room offer insights into how the first 1,000 days idea came to be part of everyday understandings of health and life. I attended the clinic with my participants for their antenatal and postnatal follow-up visits. Obtaining one's folder, having measurements taken, and finally seeing the nurse was a stepwise process that often took the better part of a day. As the study participants and I passed the time with conversation, we often talked about clinic services. The participants were highly aware of the concepts illustrated by clinic staff, health promoters, posters, and pamphlets, and these concepts circulated among the women, particularly during waiting time.

Lindiwe related the story of the long wait at her two-month clinic visit. "There's always a nurse standing there mos [obviously] when you are waiting, telling us we must breastfeed," she told me. While Lindiwe herself was not following this advice, she relished describing how she had admonished the woman next to her in the queue for not doing so, based on the impression that her infant was overweight. "It's too much [formula milk]!" she exclaimed, "She will go to the day hospital for the rest of her life!" Lindiwe was concerned that the infant was already overweight and that overfeeding the child with infant formula might increase the risk of childhood illnesses such as asthma and later-life diseases, most notably diabetes.

Inam similarly linked early complementary feeding to later obesity: "There's nothing wrong with being on a schedule for the baby to eat. Not every time they cry you make a cereal and then feed them. Because then they just want bigger portions, they get bigger and bigger, and you have an obese child at age five. No: I like proper food, prepared in a certain way. If you get fat on junk, you're not fit. Then you get high blood or diabetes. And all these things could have been avoided." She planned to start her baby on complementary foods between four and six months: "I like a certain lifestyle. I want that lifestyle for him too. I'll start him on veg. Not cereals—they're too sweet. I don't want to give him all of that sweet stuff. . . . I really want to have healthy kids, really healthy kids. If he is not meant to be a child that is going to be big, I don't want to overfeed him." She followed a website called Wholesome Foods by Momtastic for tips on what to feed him. "They say you should start with things like avocado and banana."

While Inam and Lindiwe made confident assertions about what to eat and what to feed children, Bathandwa was uncertain and conflicted about the nutritional advice doled out in the clinic. "It must be something that I long for because I come [to the clinic]. Some people take the advice because they see the danger ahead. But I don't like it when I am told what to do, because we are not the same." I offered that not everyone agreed that dietary advice should be part of medical care, but despite her reluctance to accept advice, Bathandwa insisted. "It *is* medical. The simple fact that you are there shows that there is something you are eating wrongly, or there is something you are lacking, or overdosing. The old people—they are never ill. Maybe colds or a stomach bug or something, but not really sick. It is because of what they eat. They were eating veggies, more veggies, imifino [spinach], you know, green stuff! Beans, original beans. Now we are ill. We are ill! Really. Everyone is ill. Sugar [diabetes], cancer, TB, HIV, you name it."

Bathandwa's insistence that nutrition was "a medical thing" was echoed by many of the women, as was the notion that one should eat "original" food instead of "ready-mades," "cheap brands," or "imitation foods" to avoid health issues. However, the casting of food as a medical concern and eating as medicating cannot be attributed solely to information dispensed in the clinics. Much of the primary care, surveillance, and research taking place in Khayelitsha under the banner of "global health" happened beyond the walls of the clinic, in the home.

GOVERNING THE HOME: GLOBAL HEALTH AND THE EVERYDAY

In late February 2015, Nomsa and I took Nobomi some cake for her birthday. In the middle of our festivities, we were interrupted by a knock on the door. Nobomi motioned to a man wearing a logoed T-shirt to come inside. He was followed by a team of women in the same uniform. The women introduced themselves as recruiters for a large-scale randomized controlled trial that was taking place in Cape Town. They gave a brief explanation in isiXhosa: it was a study to see what the effect on HIV prevalence would be if people started antiretroviral therapy as soon as possible. The study was being conducted in Khayelitsha, Delft, Wellington, and Paarl in a total of eight clinics. The funders were "Stellenbosch University and Bill Gates", they said. A team member with an electronic device for recording data proceeded with a list of questions about who lives in the house. Nobomi replied that there were nine people: her mother, who was in her 50s; her sisters, aged 28 and 17; her brothers, aged 26 and 19; and the children, aged 14, 2, and 3 months. The recruiter asked Nobomi to complete a "locator form" with contact details and she did so with her baby on her lap. The whole process was very efficient. The professional nurse arrived and explained to Nobomi that she would be taking blood. While the nurse set up her kit, questions from the recruiter continued.

"What is your level of education?"
"Grade eleven," Nobomi answered.

"Do you go to church?"
"Yes."

"Do you smoke?"
"No."

"Do you work?"
"No."

The questioning stopped momentarily as the nurse drew blood. Nobomi handed the baby to Nomsa and stretched out her arm for the tourniquet. "Just a prick, dear," the nurse said brusquely. She put some of Nobomi's blood in a vacutainer in her cooler bag. She then pricked Nobomi's finger for the rapid HIV test. There was no counseling before the test, but Nobomi was asked for her permission to test for HIV and she was asked to sign a consent form. Then the questioning continued.

"Where do you have friends?"
"Mostly here in my area."

"How many bedrooms are there in the house?"
"Three."

"Do you have electricity?"
"Yes."

The HIV rapid test took some minutes. I asked if they only tested for HIV and the recruiter responded that they also tested for hepatitis B and syphilis. I asked how they choose their participants. She explained that they randomize by household. "You must do one person in each household." I noticed that they were not interested in Nobomi's brother, who kept walking in and out of the lounge. I asked how they chose who in the household would participate. "We do the head of the household," said the recruiter. The nurse interjected and corrected her: they are supposed to randomize from all of the eligible participants in the house. Conveniently, the computer's randomization of household members meant that Nobomi was the one to be recruited. I asked Nobomi if this was her first study and she said no; she had been involved in a study on tuberculosis in the previous year and had been paid 500 rand for her involvement.[5] The nurse, who was waiting for the rapid test result, was unimpressed. "They make money, my dear. We are just the data collectors, the ground workers. They are sitting in an office, and they'll make the bucks. When the media asks, their name will be there—Professor so and so. My name won't be on anything." The nurse expressed frustration about doing the work "that makes the study run" without any recognition. And then they were off, breezing out as fast as they had breezed in. I said hurriedly as they left that I'd noted down everything that had happened and might describe it elsewhere but would anonymize the name of the trial and the researchers. The nurse smiled and said, "No problem."

This vignette illustrates the "everydayness" of research participation in Khayelitsha: global health forms and actors are present in all kinds of spaces and inhabit layers of intimate life. Global health projects arrive in homes and interrupt the cutting of a birthday cake or the feeding of a child. The vignette also reveals my own awkward insertion into the scene: although it was Nobomi's birthday, she was very happy to accept both the ethnographer's offer to share a small celebration and the trial team's interruptions of her birthday party.

The normalcy of trial recruitment for people living in the township might be thought of as part of the paradigm of "experimentality" that has been described for contemporary practices of global health in African life (Nguyen 2010). As Adriana Petryna (2009, 2) has noted in her extensive work on clinical trials, "trial participation becomes a form of mainstream medicine" for those who might not otherwise have access to quality care. In Nobomi's household, the family had an inside track. Her mother worked as a research assistant and referred her adult children to studies that might come with some benefits. Nobomi's experience echoes other anthropological work with clinical trial participants in South Africa, which reports that participants enroll with the understanding that they will personally benefit (Stadler et al. 2008; Cousins and Reynolds 2014). Eirik Saethre and Jonathan Stadler's study (2017) of an HIV prevention trial in Gauteng showed that for some participants, trials also afford an opportunity to perform a moral subjectivity as altruists contributing to research. A trial might also offer a break from the boredom of sitting at home doing nothing (Stadler et al. 2015; Stadler et al. 2008), a sentiment echoed by some of my participants, who quickly tired of watching TV, napping, or cleaning the house. For Nobomi, her trial involvement reassured her that she did not have cancer or tuberculosis. Some gave her access to HIV tests once a year without visiting the clinic. "I like studies," she said. "It is good for me. If there is a sickness going on in me, I will know." She told me that she took part in other studies because she was given supermarket vouchers or cash for her time. This was Nobomi's fifth clinical trial.

I am not the first to be concerned about the need to consider the everyday in relation to clinical trial participation. Working in Burkina Faso, Charlotte Brives (2013) has worked to reconnect trial participation to everyday experiences and to explore how it affects people's lives, relationships, and understandings of health care. Geissler and colleagues (2008) have written about the forms of relational ethics that structure engagements between fieldworkers and participants in The Gambia and the ambivalent familiarity that arises as long-term research produces, in essence, a "trial family" of researchers and participants. Justin Dixon (2012, 43) has also noted the "ordinariness" of trial teams in South Africa doing their door-to-door visits, developing a "nurtured degree of familiarity." Like Stadler and colleagues, Dixon witnessed a willingness among participants to engage with research teams, who for some were clearly delivering a form of care, alongside the experiment.

The households I came to be a part of during fieldwork were visited by trial recruitment teams, nongovernmental outreach services, community health care workers, and even shady salesmen hoping to sell products with perceived health benefits. I came to understand that for these households, this was a normal and expected part of life in Khayelitsha. Although Nobomi welcomed such visits and saw them as resources, not all of my participants felt the same way. Nonyameko's experience is illustrative.

Carrying the Scale

During one of the afternoons we spent with Nonyameko shortly after her baby's birth, our conversation was interrupted by "Nqo nqo!" (Knock knock!) at the door of the zinc shack she shared with some friends. Two women wearing uniform shirts with a small logo of mother and child over the left breast introduced themselves. "I am the mentor mother for this lady," the first one explained. They had come to weigh the baby and clean the umbilical cord as part of the program they ran with pregnant women they had met in the clinic or in the community. If the baby was not gaining weight sufficiently, the mother was referred to the program's nutrition advisor, who could "teach the mother how to eat and how to feed the baby," the mentor mother explained.

She put down her backpack and unpacked rubbing alcohol, some cotton swabs, and her scale. Her instructions and explanations were efficient and businesslike as she went about her tasks. She set the scale down on the makeshift floor—a carpet laid over the sandy dunes—and explained that she needed to calibrate it first. She demonstrated how to zero the scale and checked that it was working by weighing herself first. As she stood on the scale, a warning light flashed on the screen.

"Is it working?" I asked her.

"Yes, it is working, but the floor is not level," she said.

She picked up the scale, moved it to the other end of the room and started the process again. This time she managed to calibrate the scale and read her weight: 90 kilograms (198 pounds). She nodded and asked Nonyameko to hand her the baby. She weighed the baby by holding her while standing on the scale again and then subtracting her weight from the total. "4.2 kilograms" (9.25 pounds). She recorded this in a Croxley A4 notebook. After a rapid exchange in isiXhosa with Nonyameko, she packed up her scale and equipment and bade us a good day.

The mentor mothers had met Nonyameko during the last trimester of her pregnancy. Ever since, they had visited periodically without making prior arrangements. They would visit antenatally, then three days after birth, then at one week, at one month, and then monthly. "The problem is that when they come, they are not phoning," Nonyameko exclaimed, "so it is not a good idea. This is not my house. It's not good at all—you should phone and ask. They don't give you a choice." She contrasted this with our time with her. We had always phoned to make advance arrangements at a convenient time for her, and the option was available for her to tell us that she didn't want to see us anymore. "They don't say 'if you like.'" She seemed distressed after this visit. The mentor mother was not pleased to hear about Nonyameko's plan to leave Khayelitsha to return to the Eastern Cape and also disapproved of Nonyameko's decision to start formula feeds. "She doesn't know the situation," Nonyameko said.

The mentor mother organization's website stresses that "if you get the first 1000 days (including gestation) right your impact over the life course of a child is much easier; you get it wrong and you're playing catch up." During pregnancy, the mentor mothers monitored a woman's weight and, after the birth, the weight and well-being of her infant. "The scale is an important tool in getting entry into a household," the website explains. "Mothers are keen to weigh their children and the scale becomes the central point around which a discussion about child nutrition and health takes place."

From my participants' perspectives, the arrival of a trial team, a mentor mother, an NGO, or a community health care worker was either an opportunity with potential rewards for participation or a frequent and unwanted intrusion that was nevertheless tolerated as part of everyday life in the township. At the same time, mentor mothers are from the same community and often use their work to navigate this landscape. The contradictions of simultaneously being a "mentor mother" and a pregnant woman or parent became apparent in an interview with Zola, herself pregnant and previously a mentor mother, and her colleague Cebisa, who continued to work for the NGO.

Cebisa explained how the program worked: "We are mentor mothers. We receive the list of mothers from the clinic and then we follow them and make sure that they have booked [enrolled for antenatal care]. Even if we don't have the list, if you see someone who is pregnant, you ask them if they have booked. Then we follow each and every thing after that." She outlined their tasks, including discussing HIV testing, monitoring the baby after birth, checking the umbilical cord, promoting breastfeeding, and assessing the infant's weight gain. "We carry our own scales. Tape measures, surgical spirits [rubbing alcohol], gloves, tools, everything, so we just go and visit. If she is three months [pregnant], we visit her monthly. If she is six, it is fortnightly and when she is eight months, it is each and every week, because anything can happen then." I asked how many households they visited. Zola and Cebisa told me that they needed to see fifteen households each per day—a heavy schedule—to earn the stipend offered by the NGO: about 1,000 rand per month.[6] Zola and Cebisa relied on this income to support their families. "My little stipend is doing everything at home," Zola said. She supported her younger siblings and her own children. Cebisa wanted to finish her schooling but needed to support her six-year-old daughter. "With what I get I must buy winter clothes, summer clothes, she must go to school, the food that we eat! I must work hard. I must carry that scale every day." Cebisa said she didn't want to "end up here," working for little pay, carrying the scale every day. Zola described herself as "retrenched" from the NGO in the past few months. For these women, the work they did was not "volunteering," as the NGO frames it, but a form of poorly paid and insecure employment.

As Ramah McKay (2018a) has described in her work on Mozambique, the community labor NGO staff perform is central to projects of global health, and community workers or volunteers frequently occupy an ambiguous role in which they perceive themselves as both carers and wage earners in their community work. McKay also observed the ambiguities of the medical and relational labor that such workers perform. In Nobomi's case, the trial team operated in a biomedical register that included asking for her consent to participate before they proceeded. In Nonyameko's case, the mentor mothers who followed up did not ask for consent. Rather, they assumed an authority that sanctioned their visits, an authority that one might argue is legitimized by a normative understanding that traverses the state, NGOs, and the community that the mother-child dyad is "dependent" and in need of surveillance.

Surveying the Social

Seated in a large glass-walled cafeteria at the medical school, two public health registrars[7] explained their new pilot project to me: a maternal and child health screening tool that would use household-level community surveillance to assess vulnerability and offer referrals as appropriate. I wanted to learn more about the pilot and had said that I might have helpful insights for the project's design given my fieldwork experience in Khayelitsha. But the senior registrar did not want to run the pilot there. "There's so much going on in Khayelitsha," he said. That was true. Would another set of community health care workers be welcome, given that households in Khayelitsha are already covered by trial recruitment teams, mentor mothers, census recorders, door-to-door salesmen of "health" products, and more? The registrars agreed that the pilot would take place in another low-income area of Cape Town. The idea was to do an "assessment of vulnerability" for each household and complete a household registration that would record general information such as the level of household income and the education level of household members. However, the registrars disagreed about how to register people. The senior doctor preferred to use a national identity number that would be consistent across government agencies. His colleague wanted to set up a centralized data collection system that would enable a health care worker to collect and view a wealth of information about issues such as immunization checks, tuberculosis screens, compliance with medication, and records from social workers related to grant access or substance abuse. I agreed with the senior registrar that this second option was too ambitious and too difficult to implement given that the government classifies programs as part of either health services or social services. The proposal, the senior doctor said, would focus on a set of measurable items related to maternal and child health—something that would be "sustainable." He conceded that this focus had a downside: "Men are really pushed off the edge . . . really excluded from the net of the program." He concluded that the end goal of the program would be the ongoing assessment of all households by community health workers, effectively turning the home into a satellite site for the clinic. The disagreement between the registrars introduces a question: of what falls within the remit of health and how far that remit might extend into the social.

During the course of my fieldwork, I came to understand how global ideas about nutrition during the perinatal period made their way through policy channels, NGO campaigns, and the media to land in makeshift dwellings built on sandy dunes where a scale must contend with the uneven floor. It would be easy to cast the presence of foreign research teams as "neocolonial," the clinic's counsel as a neoliberal prescription for personal responsibility for one's health, or the ordinariness of home visits by NGO workers as an insidious form of surveillance. I will argue that the scenes I have described do not offer such ready diagnoses. Rather, when pieced together, these vignettes illustrate fragmentary logics that inform new forms of governance and intervention by both state and non-state actors today.

CONCEPTS OF LIFE

That focusing on pregnant women and children "gets you somewhere" with both state structures and private donors is a function of the perceived economic pay-offs, and of the currency of the mother-child dyad in contemporary global health on the African continent. The first 1,000 days appeals to the logics of both saving "lives" and valuing "life."

The contemporary value placed on "life," as Barbara Duden (1993, 2) has argued, is a concept most fully embodied by the unborn child. Her work on the abortion debate in twentieth-century Germany showed how "in the course of one generation, technology along with a new discourse, has transformed pregnancy into a process to be managed, the expected child into a fetus, the mother into an ecosystem, the unborn into a life, and life into a supreme value." Didier Fassin (2012a, 111), drawing on his work on the South African HIV pandemic, argues that "it is possible—and indeed crucial—to differentiate evaluations having for their object the worth of lives, and judgments predicated on the value of life. The grammatical number (lives versus life) is as important here as the lexical variation (worth versus value)."

Underpinning the first 1,000 days concept is a judgment about the value of a life, which is constituted in economic terms as "human capital" and has been newly conceived as an epigenetic outcome of early life nutrition. Human capital formation is captured in the indices of adult height, educational achievement, income, and birth weight of offspring. One can view these indicators, following Fassin (2012a), as "qualitative data offering political insights as to how societies produce and reproduce themselves" (109; see also Canguilhem 1978). Interventions in the early life period are based on an economic logic that reflects a "hard-nosed economic calculus" (Osmani and Sen 2003), an understandable rationale in an era that demands measurable economic outcomes and capital creation. In addition, pregnant and newborn populations are easy to count. In the "systematic triage" (Nguyen 2010, 178) that allocates funding and resources, a population that is easily constituted, easily singled out for intervention, and easily counted—a governable population—appeals to the measurability, reproducibility, and "scaling up" that global health projects require (Adams 2016). As a project of global health, the first 1,000 days is thus one instantiation of how the epistemology of market logics informs the life sciences and their application to public health concerns—what Kaushik Sunder Rajan (2012, 1) calls "the capitalization of life." That this capitalization now includes distant future health outcomes based on epigenetic understandings of disease transmission exemplifies Fassin's (2012a, 112) summation that there has been "a profound change in the recognition of the value of life, which has shifted from the political to the biological."

If the image of the fetus is the paradigmatic emblem of "life," the image of the African mother and child is arguably its other—the paradigmatic emblem of "lives." Despite the global remit of the concept of the first 1,000 days, the websites, posters, pamphlets, and media that promote related interventions commonly feature images of *African* women and children, many of which are reminiscent of those used to depict "Third World" famine (Burman 1994) and AIDS orphans in Africa (Fassin 2013). The deployment of the African mother-child dyad and the moral sentiment it seeks to elicit exemplifies the logic of "humanitarian government" that characterized global health in the early twenty-first century (Fassin 2012b). The contemporary circulation of this assemblage—a trope closely tied to the invention of Africa (Mudimbé 1988)—acts as a "travelling technology" (Petryna 2009; Von Schnitzler 2013) that configures contemporary global health policy. In the pamphlets that circulate through the waiting rooms in the antenatal clinics of Khayelitsha, that trope reappears in the form of a stylized image of mother and child and the message that "the first 1000 days of a child's life is a very important time for shaping a child's ability to grow and develop." In this iconography, the image of the child carries "affective authority," as Liisa Malkki (2015, 79) puts it, to constitute a transnational sphere of exchanges that can be thought of as ritual acts, given that they appear and are conceived of as "apolitical, even suprapolitical," even though they have clearly political outcomes. In Johanna Tayloe Crane's (2013) assessment, global health projects in Africa today reproduce the colonial motivations of "extraction" and "salvation" that Nancy Rose Hunt (1999) has described as the main historical concerns of empire in Africa. "Salvation," in this formulation, has no better illustration than the repetitive images of African women and their infants that accompany promotional material, donor websites, editorials, media campaigns, and the like.

MEDICALIZING THE AFRICAN "SOCIAL"

The view that "the house and domestic families are directly impinged upon by the forces of the state" (Carsten 2003, 50) has been a central feature of Foucauldian analyses of the home (Foucault 1978; Donzelot 1979). In Clara Han's (2012) ethnography of indebted Chilean households in the wake of neoliberal reforms in the early 2000s, she remarks that "rather than thinking of the forces of the state as 'impinging' on the house from without, however, we can think of multiple ways in which the state is layered in people's intimate lives" (17). In the present example, it becomes clear that it is not only the state but also a network of nonstate actors that might be collectively described as an archipelago of global health science that inhabits these layers of intimate life.

If Africa is still a "living laboratory" (Tilley 2011), its power resides in such archipelagos, which are constituted by a set of links between a local university, research center, or academic hospital; a scientific organization based in the Global North; and a European or American university, international philanthropist, or not-for-profit organization—or a combination of these (Geissler 2013b). Khayelitsha is one such island, as indicated by the sheer number of research projects that occur there. The township exemplifies the desirable trial population, characterized by "sufficient technical and bureaucratic infrastructure to run a clinical trial, with willing trial subjects motivated by poverty and a poor health care system, with motivated local research partners who depend on the income generated by this work, and with a legal system that is predictable and yet not too closely knit and rigid for the interests of research" (Rottenburg 2009, 424).

The new forms of governmentality at work—defined as the collection of technologies and means by which individuals govern themselves (Foucault 2008)—are captured by the trial and the scale. The ubiquity of the former suggests that Khayelitsha in some ways exemplifies the contemporary African biopolitical configuration of trial community and experimental society that Vinh-Kim Nguyen (2010) described as "experimentality." The presence of scales in the backpacks of NGO employees who enter people's homes is indicative of how maternal and child nutrition as a regime of knowledge and intervention is newly enfolded within the purview of governance.

The presence of the trial and the scale in the everyday in Khayelitsha could easily be glossed as a further extension of medicalization—the expansion of scientific medicine's jurisdictions into new social domains (Zola 1972)—or bio-medicalization, characterized by changed political economies, an increased biomedical focus on health surveillance and risk, technoscientific biomedical innovations, new modes of producing and consuming biomedical information, and new forms of citizenship and identity (Clarke et al. 2003). Nguyen (2015) has argued that "the social" that underpins prevailing formulations of medicalization corresponds to a Eurocentric version characterized by a contract between a nation-state and its citizens. In this world view, the shared membership of citizens in the same nation-state constitutes a common bond. This Durkheimian model has little application in African settings. For many African contexts, Nguyen states, "society" in the Durkheimian sense is fragile and thus medicalization might manifest quite differently. James Ferguson is similarly concerned with "the African social" in his work on welfare programs in southern Africa. He argues that the remit of "the social" (Durkheim [1895] 1982) and its genealogy to eventually constitute the European welfare state has little relevance in the Global South, where "neoliberal restructuring represents not a 'rolling back' of a Keynesian welfare state but the very context within which new forms of social protection have been pioneered" (Ferguson 2015, 68). Ferguson sees the realization of the "social" in southern Africa as linked to the fostering of "proper" African workers, "living in 'proper', 'European-style' nuclear families" (71; see also Ferguson 1999). This version of "the social" remains prominent, as is evidenced by the trial team's concern with where Nobomi's friends live, whether she works or not, and if she attends church.

Yet in South Africa, the "invention of the social" was premised on a logic of discrimination that extended welfare provision to inhabitants on a highly skewed and racialized scale (Ferguson 2015, 75). This is important for the present discussion given that, as Ferguson asserts, an analysis cannot start from a point of "*the* social" but must depart from "*this* social—that is, the historically particular and decidedly nonegalitarian 'social' of white settlers and black labor aristocracies in southern Africa" (77). *This* social is also one that cannot be properly understood without attention to gender: the designation of women's roles has been integral to state formation in the colonial, apartheid, and post-apartheid eras (Manicom 1992).

The "decentralization of the clinic" (Carney 2015, 198) delivers clinical authority to previously intimate—and gendered—spaces. In South Africa, the forms of medicalization that are reflected in the ordinariness of recruitment and surveillance of women are the manifestation of long histories of colonial and state intervention that have delineated what counts as "domestic" as opposed to economic or public space. These arrangements replicate long-standing gendered and racialized constructions of the place of women. In her ethnography of public sector responses to obesity in postwar Guatemala, Emily Yates-Doerr (2015a, 163) found that "metrification" was perhaps a better concept than medicalization for describing government interventions that focused on body measurements and corresponding protocols. This concept is useful for considering the centrality of the scale in the surveillance projects I observed. That these scales were not part of a state surveillance system but were carried out by NGO staff again highlights the legitimate engagement of nonstate actors in such projects, authorized by a global discourse of the mother-infant pair as "vulnerable."

The Maternal in the "Social"

The problematic normative use of the nuclear family to describe social arrangements in South Africa has long been a focus of regional scholarship (Burman and Reynolds 1986; Ramphele 1993; Spiegel et al. 1996). Ferguson argues that the nuclear family that constituted the desired social of state interventions in South Africa no longer has the cultural authority it once did. In the provision of social grants in South Africa, for example, cash transfers are given to "primary care givers"; biological kinship no longer configures welfare transactions. And yet, as Ferguson (2015) concedes, "the privileging of the mother-and-child figure as the key recipients of cash transfers [has] arguably fed a global renewal of a kind of paternalism" (41). The definition of recipients of social welfare in South Africa (and elsewhere) as persons deemed "dependent"—children, the elderly, the disabled—reveals implicit assumptions about who constitutes the economically active, "independent" population—young, able-bodied men—and thus serves a particular vision of the social in which male breadwinners support their heteronormative nuclear families.

The focus on the first 1,000 days is one reflection of this renewed paternalism, and yet in this African social, it is the maternal figure that is called upon to perform what Melinda Cooper and Catherine Waldby (2014, 13) term clinical labor: "the process of material abstraction by which the abstract, temporal imperatives of accumulation are put to work at the level of the body." They cite examples such as surrogacy, tissue donation, and participation in clinical trials. In a similar fashion, the logic of the first 1,000 days makes ordinary pregnancy and early infant care a link in the chain that creates capital.

In this chapter I have traversed different sites of the global health archipelago and have shown how domestic space (or the home) is a crucial part of this formation. Global health is not just created in universities, research centers, hospitals, and not-for-profits; it is also created in thousands of homes where clinical trial participants are recruited. The ordinariness of trial participation for people living in Khayelitsha is indicative of the spatializing effects of global health. It is not sufficient to go out and study "other spaces of global health" (Herrick 2017); rather, we need to be aware of how global health configures space and the routes such configurations take (Povinelli 2011). Ordinary spaces are vital for the global health project, but they are constituted and configured by spatialized histories. In South Africa, the distinct history of spatialized inclusion or exclusion continues to configure the routes and flows of people, capital, and technologies that make the presence of a trial team in one's living room entirely ordinary in certain parts of the city while other visits that would be ordinary and expected in other parts of the city (the postman or the refuse collector) are not ordinary in Khayelitsha. Indeed, their absence is often the cause of activist protest in the township. The living room, the home, the township, and the relations that are figured through domesticity and kinship are in fact vital organs of global health— or rather, spatialized effects of relations between states, organizations, blood samples, and demographic data that require intimate forms of labor to produce the circulations and effects that go by the name of global health. For Nobomi, participation in multiple trials is simply part of the strategies she uses to continue forging life in this place; the circulation of a trial team through her living room is as everyday as her neighbor sauntering in and out of the house. Questions of boundaries of public and private space, of state and citizen, thus take on a unique configuration in South Africa given how the social is spatialized and given the role of gender in apartheid and post-apartheid state formation.

In analyzing present-day policy, an ahistorical view easily overlooks the centrality of Black women's subordination to the development and maintenance of the apartheid project and the fact that "the very fundamental categories of state and politics—like citizen, worker, the modern state itself—are shot through with gender" (Manicom 1992, 444). Just as cash transfers might reinvigorate older forms of paternalism in South Africa, trial participation is configured by particular norms, gender roles, and expectations. Trial protocols might describe recruiting "individuals" who are sharing a "household" by a process of randomization, but it was not surprising in Nobomi's case that it was she the team selected rather than her adult brother. How domestic space is integrated into the archipelago is shaped by local histories—in this case, of migrant labor systems during apartheid that left a legacy of female-headed households and split families—and of a more recent history of HIV and the configuration of the pregnant woman as a key trial participant.

The politics of potential expresses a powerful biological framework for the value of life. In identifying the substance of potential in the vulnerable mother-child dyad, it shapes the delivery of health care and legitimizes forms of governance and self-governance in clinical and domestic spheres. In the next chapter, I focus on how this logic shapes the implementation of clinical care and the implications of that for the problem of responsibility.

4 · LIFE BETWEEN PROTOCOLS

It is a windy September morning in 2014 and an early start at the clinic. At the gate, a vendor unpacks sweets, chips, and fruit for people to purchase before they join the queue. There is a Médecins Sans Frontières vehicle in the parking lot. The queue starts well before the 8 a.m. opening time. Once the door has swung open, a security guard waves people through to reception. Patients request their folders and take a seat on the plastic chairs that fill the large waiting area. The space frequently fills up so that patients stand all along the windows and the walls, and the room murmurs with the low rumble of conversations and the shuffling of feet. In the entrance hall, a large noticeboard is filled with a series of posters on Ebola that use cartoons to explain Ebola's symptoms and prevention:

"Ebola, don't catch it! You can catch Ebola from someone who is sick or dead. Keep away . . ."

"EBOLA is in animals and bats too. DO NOT touch or eat bush meat and don't eat bats."

"Ebola: What is it? Ebola is caused by a virus. Causes a severe illness with bleeding. Up to 90% will die. No vaccine and no treatment are available. Many people can quickly become infected."

"WASH YOUR HANDS OFTEN. Use SOAP. DON'T TOUCH! Do not touch an infected person or their body fluids."

Nomsa and I weave our way through the bustling reception, where patients are shoulder to shoulder and trying to make out their names as they are called out on the loudspeaker. The clinic feels like one long congested passageway, with little seating for patients. Everything is slightly worn, but mostly clean. We step into the children's observation room—a tiny office filled with parents and their babes in arms. The heater is on, the window is closed, and the room feels stuffy. There is no nursing sister present. Further down the corridor, we find the Tuberculosis room, and then just outside, a small zinc container, with a large plaque and a USAID logo that reads: "The United States President's Emergency Plan for AIDS Relief. The Power of Partnerships. This project is proudly supported by the American people through PEPFAR." We find Sr. Josephs after some enquiries, and I introduce myself as a researcher from the University of Oxford. She responds, "Oh, from the States." I correct her and she is surprised to hear that I've come from a British institution and not an American one, noting the frequency with which students from the United States pass through the clinic.

—Field notes, September 10, 2014

Even though South Africa and all of southern Africa remained free of Ebola infection during the 2014 outbreak, the spectacle of the outbreak and the global health response to it was evident, alongside the long-standing global health programs for HIV and tuberculosis care. Stickers on seating, posters on walls and doors, and stationery in consulting rooms bearing the logos of USAID, the US President's Emergency Plan for AIDS Relief (PEPFAR), and Médecins Sans Frontières, among others, were evidence of the global health actors that worked in conjunction with state facilities in primary care clinics. Organizations such as Médecins Sans Frontières had a visible staff presence in clinical settings, where they recruited patients for some of their programs. On an average weekday, one would inevitably meet one of the many groups of American students from prestigious US universities who had come to Cape Town to take part in a "research collaboration" as part of their global health training (see also Crane 2013).

The materials and rhetoric of "global health" at the clinic mainly exhorted people to take personal responsibility to prevent infectious diseases. In contrast with the logic of pandemic preparedness, nutrition policy focused on the first 1,000 days exhorted mothers to take personal responsibility for the future health of their babies as part of a politics of potential that reflects the specific configuration of state, science, and citizens in South Africa. In this chapter, I explore the inherent contradictions in this politics and the resulting disjunctures between protocol and practice. On paper, protocol-driven care fits into linear diagrams. In reality, it must contend with bodies that do not neatly conform to categories. Protocol sidelines context in ways that produce moral injury for health care practitioners and it is subject to improvisation on the part of staff when tools fail or when time is short. In reality, protocol must bend and flow through fixed material infrastructures that contain both gestures toward imagined futures and residues of the past.

DESIGN AND AFFECT

In South Africa, the clinic does not share the dominant historical narrative of colonial and postcolonial medicine that exists elsewhere on the continent. The enactment of global health in South Africa rests on a far more recent history of nation-building and of a public health sector irrevocably shaped by the HIV pandemic. As one clinic manager explained, the setup of clinics in South Africa were frequently the outcome of "historic processes rather than a rational plan."

I conducted fieldwork at the Kunye Clinic and the Sunrise Clinic, the former a few years older than the latter. The difference in clinic design and layout between these two spaces was testimony to the changing history of primary health care provision in South Africa and the integration of HIV management into public sector service provision. The design of the Kunye Clinic—a brick-faced U-shaped building with a central courtyard—was like that of many of the older clinics of Cape Town where I had worked as a clinician. Patients entered one end of the U for the reception and waiting area, then proceeded to consult-ing rooms located along either side of the corridor, and then to the health educa-tion waiting area and the pharmacy before exiting. Consulting rooms in the building were divided into four categories: adults, children, tuberculosis patients, and antenatal care. The tuberculosis room was directly adjacent to the antenatal rooms and the patients waited alongside one another to be seen. HIV services were provided in zinc prefab structures sponsored by PEPFAR that were located outside of and apart from the clinic building. This meant that although there was a clinical mandate to integrate general and HIV services, in practice patients were still required to circulate through more than one consultation room before heading to the "temporary" PEPFAR containers outside.

The design and flow of the Sunrise Clinic avoided some of the problems of such a setup. At the entrance, patients were directed to what staff termed the "infectious" side for HIV and tuberculosis care services on the right or to the "chronic" side for antenatal, pediatric, adult, and wellness services on the left. According to clinic doctors, the "adult chronics" had conditions such as hyperten-sion, diabetes, and osteoarthritis. The wellness clinic served HIV-positive patients who were not yet on antiretroviral therapy. Patient flow proceeded in a similar fashion to the setup at the Kunye Clinic, from the large reception/waiting area where patients retrieved their folders to the observations room to smaller waiting areas where health promotion sessions were delivered in a consulting room, and finally to the pharmacy to collect medication. The difference was that the possi-bility of tuberculosis exposure for patients was minimized, although the arrange-ment at Sunrise still meant that HIV services were not fully integrated into general primary care. At the entrance to each clinic there was a map to guide patients. At Kunye, it was a hand-drawn sketch, and at Sunrise, it was a laminated, profession-ally printed diagram—a difference that hints at some of the other material differ-ences between the two clinics.

These differences in clinic design and aesthetics had an impact on the experi-ences of both staff and patients. That is to say, the clinic itself was what Alice Street (2012, 45) refers to as an "affective technology". In her ethnography of a hospital in Papua New Guinea, Street (2014, 21) argues that hospitals (and clinics) need to be understood "as historical as well as spatial infrastructures." Street (2012) showed how the layered histories of postcolonial buildings and the materialities of doing health care work produce affective spaces of both hope and resignation.

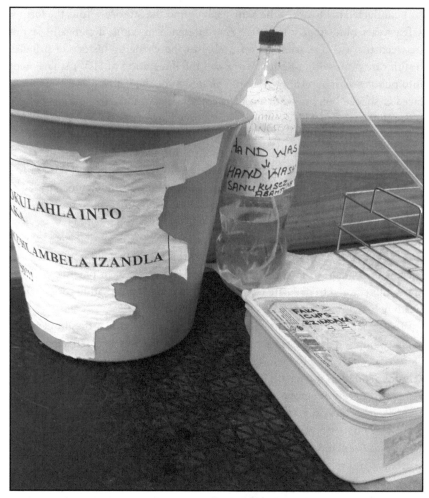

FIGURE 7. The oral rehydration station at Sunrise Clinic, including a makeshift tap (inverted Coca-Cola bottle) for handwashing, a bucket of fresh water and an ice cream tub of a mixture of sugar and salt for making up the oral rehydration solution (6 teaspoons of sugar and half a teaspoon of salt per 1 liter of water). (Photographed by the author, November 2014)

Khayelitsha's clinics conjured expectations of the nation and of modernity. Bright yellow posters adorned Sunrise clinic's walls, advertising the City of Cape Town as the 2014 World Design Capital. In the staff room, a poster quoted Nelson Mandela: "It always seems impossible until it is done." The tagline: "African innovation. Global conversation." In the wellness clinic, another poster quoted Steve Jobs: "Design is not just what it looks like. Design is how it works." The tagline: "Beautiful spaces, beautiful things." And in the observations area, a poster quoted a Chinese proverb: "The best time to plant a tree was twenty years ago. The next best time is today." Below: "Today for Tomorrow." The presence of World Design Capital posters throughout the clinic stamped this space as part of the city's future-making project. Yet people often sat in broken chairs in the waiting room. Older posters with curled edges had been repaired with patient identification stickers. Oral rehydration stations in waiting rooms consisted of an old Coca-Cola bottle converted into a container for handwashing, a bucket of fresh water, and an ice-cream tub filled with the rehydration mixture of sugar and salt (Figure 7). *Design is not just what it looks like and feels like. Design is how it works.*

In the Kunye and Sunrise clinics, antenatal care offices contained an old wooden desk and an examination table. Each desk had a calendar, a body mass index wheel, a dating wheel to aid in the quick calculation of fetal gestational age, and a heap of paperwork—lab results, protocols, and diaries. As was the case in most public clinics in Cape Town at that time, notes were still made with pen and paper. The examination area was equipped with a blood pressure cuff, a light, a tape measure, examination gloves, disinfectant, lubricant jelly, and a plastic feto-scope, a hollow trumpet-shaped device used to listen to fetal heartbeats. Designed by French obstetrician Adolphe Pinard in the nineteenth century, the device has been largely replaced by Doppler ultrasound in high-income countries and in the private sector in South Africa. Although the fetoscope remains an important and effective tool for midwifery in primary care in South Africa, its use did not go unnoticed by patients. "I know this is not a private hospital," Lindiwe told me one day in the waiting room, "but I'd be happier if they could do a few scans." Pregnant women hoped to experience an ultrasound scan, but this was mostly unavailable in the public sector. The clinic was thus an affective space of both nostalgia and futurity (see also Street 2012; Geissler and Lachenal 2016). Expectations of modernity embedded in the materiality of the metropolitan clinic made it a site of ambivalence for those who inhabited it, especially when their expectations were not met.

PRACTICES OF MEASUREMENT

A child, two pregnant women, and an elderly gentleman are crowded around the scales, and the sister directs each to take their turn. There is an old balance scale and a digital scale with a large Médecins Sans Frontières sticker on its face. The child is instructed to take off her sandals and she removes them clumsily. She is weighed and her height is measured against the wall. The sister taps the scale forcefully with her foot to recalibrate it and the first woman steps forward. The sister does not ask her to remove her shoes. The woman is weighed with her folder in her hand. Next, the elderly man has removed his shoes, but not his bulky overcoat. The nurse instructs him to take it off and he drapes it over the balance scale and stands on the digital one. The second woman also wears an overcoat and is weighed in it without comment. The nurse writes the measurements in black ink on each patient's hands—weight on the right, height on the left. For smaller children, their measurements are written on their mothers' hands. These numbers will be recorded in the folder once the patient enters the observations room for blood pressure and glucose measurements.

—Excerpt from field notes, September 16, 2014

At the Sunrise Clinic, a nurse supervised the weighing of patients on a digital scale or a balance scale in the waiting area. The nurse would weigh everyone in the waiting room in about fifteen minutes and then return when a new group of patients had arrived to repeat the exercise. The stratification of pregnant women into two groups—one deemed eligible for therapeutic nutrition supplementation and the other for lifestyle and nutrition counseling—rested on the practice of measuring height, weight, and mid-upper arm circumference (MUAC). At the Kunye Clinic, adult patients would weigh themselves on a digital scale in the waiting area and report the number to the nurse when they reached the observations room. "You must weigh yourself, then you say 'I weigh this weight,'" Aviwe explained to me. "You could say anything to those nurses," she laughed, "seventy kilograms instead of fifty kilograms!"

I frequently witnessed the ritual of the scale, and I was most struck by the inconsistency with which the nurse would request that jackets, shoes, overcoats, and folders be set aside before stepping on the scale. There was little or no standardization in the way this measurement was taken, even though its purpose was to enable stratification and intervention according to an agreed-upon standard. This was not because consistency was not possible due to a lack of resources or lack of knowledge. Rather, observing the ritual of the scale was an exercise in recognizing the ethical, which comes into view with "close attention to *the actual conduct* of life in the world" (Lambek 2015, 11, emphasis in original). Nurses deviated from the technoscientific script (Akrich 1992), perhaps because they were disaffected with their task or perhaps because they were attending to another social script that accorded respect to some categories of persons. Having observed the ritual of the scale many times, I suggest that for the nurse, the task of weighing patients did not appear to *matter*, or at least not all of the time. Practices of measurement, in this case, undermined rather than aided the success of protocol.

On one occasion, a teenage girl was subjected to the public weighing. Others in the waiting room made jibes, like "Sjoe! [Wow!] You look fat but you're still young, why don't you try to go to a gym or get some exercise every morning?" While some fatness was considered desirable by many, being "too fat" connoted laziness. Both men and women in the waiting room commented among one another and laughed at the teenager. "150 kilograms!" Thus, it was not just the protocol of stratifying patients for nutrition supplementation that was undercut here. Also at stake in the queue for the scale and the routine inscription of numbers on hands were the fine lines between dignity and indignity, between accountability and disregard. Such practices of marking the body have uncomfortable resonances with earlier colonial attempts to enumerate and classify populations (Breckenridge 2014). If such tensions appeared in ordinary practices of measurement, they were far more pronounced in decision-making, program implementation, and evaluation in these clinics.

"THINGS ARE WRITTEN IN PROTOCOLS": HIV AND INFANT FEEDING POLICIES

Promoting breastfeeding is a key tenet of first 1,000 days policy. The policy change on infant feeding for the prevention of mother-to-child transmission (PMTCT) of HIV in the Western Cape—supporting exclusive breastfeeding and discontinuing the free provision of infant formula—came into effect some months into my time in the clinics. I was thus able to document how institutions and individuals responded to the new directive. My conversations with Sr. Qoma, who had been involved with the PMTCT program for some time, and Mrs. Tshabalala, one of the health promoters,[1] offer two accounts of how health care workers experienced the changes in PMTCT policy in the Western Cape—from exclusive formula feeding to a choice between exclusive formula and exclusive breastfeeding and finally to the policy recommendation of exclusive breastfeeding for all women regardless of HIV status.

Offering a Choice

During an initial interview with me, Sr. Qoma was at pains to emphasize the importance of the choice that was available to pregnant mothers when the policy still offered options. She explained:

> In the old days, we used to say that the PMTCT mothers are not allowed to breastfeed, but these days they are free to breastfeed as long they stick to the procedure. We tell the breastfeeding mothers: if they are positive, they can breastfeed as much as they want but they must give Bactrim daily.[2] If she can't breastfeed according to her circumstances, it is her choice, and we provide formula for those mothers here in our clinics. They make their own choices: we are not allowed.

I asked her if anyone who requested the formula could obtain it. She responded:

> No, not just anyone who requests because there are mothers that made their choice that they are going to breastfeed, ne [is it not so]? But as the time goes, they suddenly stop breastfeeding and they expect that we are going to give the formula.

The rule is not working like that—you must stick to the choice that you made while you were pregnant. And when we give them their choices we don't say to the mothers "Tell us today," we give them time to think about the choices, ne? Those months that the mothers are pregnant is their time to think: what will they feed their babies? But now the milk is no longer given in other provinces—it's only the Western Cape Department of Health still doing that, and they will change it. There will be specific people who will get milk, if the doctors say you cannot breastfeed due to certain circumstances, something like that, terminal stage or full-blown AIDS mothers cannot breastfeed—so only them, they can get the milk.

Mrs. Tshabalala similarly emphasized choice but also mentioned the AFASS criteria[3] that were used in assessing the suitability of formula feeding in the old policy:

> The feeding option—it is their choice, ne? But it is very important to explain to them, okay, exclusive breastfeeding goes like this: it is a package on its own. And the exclusive formula feeding: there are the AFASS criteria, whereby you have to see if it is feasible, affordable . . . and what is it? Sustainable and safe. All those five. Fine. If maybe a lady is staying in a squatter camp, there is no water there, you are sharing one tap, there's no electricity, you have to use the flame, this person is not working. . . . If there are those challenges, you are not qualified by AFASS criteria. Then it is her choice, she needs to say okay, I'm going to breastfeed no matter what.

In other words, if patients did not qualify for formula, they had to "choose" breastfeeding. But soon the government would not be offering formula at all. "Now there is a new protocol," Mrs. Tshabalala noted. "Things are written in protocols, ne?"

I asked her about women who may have used formula in a first pregnancy and were now pregnant again and were disappointed to find that it was no longer available. She responded:

> So it is really confusing for them, yes? But at the clinic we can say "Okay, now that you are pregnant, we are going according to a new protocol, so you have to handle the situation in this way, now, ne?" Because everybody now is encouraged to breastfeed because the treatment—you have to take it no matter if your CD4 count is high.[4] Even if a mother's CD4 count is so high that she is not on ARVs [antiretrovirals], for the sake of the child that woman has to take that pill to protect the child.

While the nurses did not demonstrate a clear understanding of the rationale behind the policy changes, they affirmed that they had received a new directive.

Sara Nieuwoudt and Lenore Manderson (2018), who interviewed frontline health care workers in Soweto in 2015–2016, have made similar observations: that health care workers were not given adequate information about these policy changes and that this produced confusion. During this conversation with Mrs. Tshabalala, I was thinking of Aviwe, whose account of the changed infant feeding policy reveals the confusion and frustration that can accompany "going according to a new protocol."

During her first pregnancy, in 2009, Aviwe learned that she was HIV positive and followed the PMTCT program at that time. She fed her first baby formula and he tested negative. She started on lifelong antiretrovirals in 2011 and had an undetectable viral load in 2014 when she found out that she was pregnant again. This time, though, the PMTCT counselors told her that she should exclusively breastfeed. She recalled how she was sent to a PMTCT counselor without any explanation from the clinic sister:

> They take you to what they call the counselors. When I was there, I asked the counselor, "Why am I here?" The counselor said, "Didn't the sister tell you?" I said, "No, she didn't tell me, but she said I must come to you. I ask you now why am I here." She said, "Yhu [wow], it's a big question. You are supposed to ask the sister. Sisi [Sister], if you don't feel like you can be here, there's no point." Then she asked me "Sisi, are you gonna breastfeed the baby?" I said no. She asked me why. I said, "No, I don't trust this thing of breastfeeding while you are positive." And she said to me, "Why do you not trust it? Your CD4—ntoni ntoni [what-what], your HIV level is right—it is LDL [lower than detectable level], we can't see anything, the viral load is low." So she said to me, "No, you are going to breast-feed this baby because what we notice now, is that you positive people don't want to breastfeed, because of this milk government is giving you." And I said to her, "No sister, it is not about that. The problem is that I have never heard anyone that said *I was breastfeeding. My child is negative. It's 100%.* I have never . . . so I don't want to take a risk. My first baby, I didn't breastfeed him, I just gave him the bottle. So he is negative. So I don't want to risk." I told her I would go and ask my husband as well. When I came back, they asked me again, and I said "My husband said he doesn't want me to breastfeed because he doesn't trust this." She laughed at me. "Wahaha! This is my first time hearing this—*my husband doesn't want me*—does it depend on your husband or does it depend on you?" I gave them the report mos [obviously]. They asked "Who's gonna buy the milk?" I said "I'm gonna see what I can do. I'm gonna buy the milk." They said, "You won't get the milk [from us] because you don't have the virus, the virus is small in your body. You're gonna answer there to those sisters why you don't want to breastfeed. Because that's not a reason. If your husband doesn't understand you should have told him to come and hear what is a risk, what is not a risk." My husband says he doesn't trust that. If you are infected, you can also infect the baby. He is scared. I

am also scared. And I said to her, the reason why I don't want to breastfeed is that I am working, and I must leave the baby. And I can't say "Don't give this baby water, don't give food, don't give what-what. Just give breast milk." Then the nanny feeds my baby. Then the milk is finished before I come back. What is she going to do? It is obvious. She is going to make a bottle. Because I am not back yet and the baby is crying. So that is the problem. She's gonna mix. So that is why I choose to just feed with a bottle. So that I can just give the nanny milk so that if I come later, there is no problem, she can just feed my baby, you see? It's not right, this "you're gonna breastfeed, Sisi, until your baby is six months."

Aviwe's experience highlights the common difficulties of HIV-positive pregnant women faced with another change in infant feeding policy. Aviwe was highly aware of the increased risk that mixed feeding posed for HIV transmission (Coutsoudis et al. 1999). Those who had pregnancies during the policy's previous incarnation and fed their infants with formula have personal proof that this method worked to prevent mother-to-child transmission. At that time, the risks and benefits of breastfeeding versus formula feeding were presented to them, framed in a discourse of personal choice and personal acknowledgment of the risks that accompanied the option they chose. As Nkululeko Nkomo (2015, 163) has discussed for PMTCT antiretroviral access in South Africa, a focus on affording women a right to choose was part of a larger rights-based discourse mobilized by HIV activists who "recast a sense of hopelessness into self-responsibilization, which concurrently involved nourishing hope in the preferred future for women with HIV to be afforded the right to individual choice associated with self-determination." In this history, it is the pregnant woman who has "the right to healthcare, autonomy and hope" (163). Given that context, it is easy to understand how the removal of choice about infant feeding was received not as a newly calibrated, apolitical scientific recommendation but rather as an affront to the self-governance cultivated in HIV discourse in South Africa as "an ideal personal and ethical quality of HIV-positive subjectivity" (167).

The new Western Cape policy directive on exclusive feeding regardless of HIV status was issued on April 2, 2015 (Circular 57 of 2015). It stipulated that as of April 1, 2015, no new HIV-positive mothers would receive infant formula with the exception of women who had been on second- or third-line antiretrovirals for three months or longer and still had a viral load that exceeded 1,000 copies per milliliter. I received this email on April 10, 2015, from my contacts in the Department of Health. Sr. Qoma later told me that the new policy was communicated to clinic staff on April 23 but that she had not received her own copy of the policy document yet and that she would wait for the formal written directive. Sr. Qoma's assertion that only the formal written directive was authoritative meant that she could continue to supply her patients with formula for as long as possible.

THE NUTRITION THERAPEUTIC PROGRAM

The 2013 Western Cape protocols for basic antenatal care (Western Cape Government 2013) specified that BMI and MUAC should be measured at the first antenatal visit using the BMI wheel and the MUAC tape distributed to clinics. A Nutrition Directorate officer explained the Nutrition Therapeutic Program to me: BMI was used as an indicator of obstetric risk, whereas MUAC provided a way to stratify women's nutritional status according to the new nutrition policy focus on the first 1,000 days.[5] A BMI greater than 30 warranted referral to the district hospital, one greater than 40 but less than 50 a referral to a regional hospital, and one greater than 50 a referral to tertiary level care. The policy specified that those classified as underweight should be referred to the Nutrition Therapeutic Program for six months of supplementation (fortified porridges, milkshakes, and peanut butter), to be taken in addition to "normal family meals" and that those who were classified as normal weight, overweight, or obese should receive dietary counseling.[6]

The directorate official was aware of some of the obstacles to the smooth implementation of the new basic antenatal care policy. "The MUAC has been done only for the past three years, so people are only getting used to it now." He was exasperated about the fact that even though the nutrition subdirectorate had provided training on how to do these measurements and distributed MUAC tape measures to all clinics, the clinical audits did not reflect that MUAC was measured consistently during antenatal visits and staff frequently reported that they did not have the tape measures. "They complain that there is just not enough time," he shrugged. The directorate had tried to streamline delivery of the nutrition package by developing a nutrition checklist with basic messages that could be ticked off so that not all of the counseling needed to be done at one visit. The official was sympathetic: "We cannot expect midwives to be generalists, but the number of dieticians is limited." He outlined the Metro Clinic arrangement: a roaming dietician visited each clinic once a month, which corroborated my observations in the clinics. Obesity, diabetes, or malnutrition warranted referral to the dietician, but in practice the staff used their discretion with referrals, which were limited by the number of cases the dietician could see in a day.

The Register

I came to understand how these policies were enacted in the clinic during an interview with Sr. Mimi at the Kunye Clinic. She explained that each clinic keeps a Nutrition Therapeutic Register, and after some shuffling of all the items on her desk, she produced the clinic's register for me. The large A3 booklet began by introducing the purpose of the register: to record "the minimum information required to monitor the implementation of the Nutrition Therapeutic Program." There were detailed instructions on how to complete entries in the register. The patient's weight and MUAC (and height or length for children) were recorded at each monthly visit. For children, each entry recorded the date of birth, birth weight, the start date of the program, and adherence to a checklist that included "vitamin A," "exclude tuberculosis," "deworm," "nutrition education," "other illnesses," and "feeding practices." Each patient was given a "category code", and the product and amount given were noted. Each patient was also assigned an "exit code" after six months on the supplementation program. Possible exit codes included:

S: *Successful*—adequate weight gain
U: *Unsuccessful*—inadequate weight gain; referral to a dietician
I: *Interrupter or Defaulter*—failure to attend the clinic, may not be reentered in
    the program without dietician's assessment
R: *Referred*—referred to the dietician before the six-month period ended
DC: *Deceased*

The clinic register that Sr. Mimi showed me had records dating back to April 2012. One- quarter of the entries in the register had an *S* exit code, indicating successful supplementation and weight gain. Three-quarters of the entries in the register had an *I* exit code, indicating that the majority of patients "interrupted" or "defaulted" from the supplementation program. I found a similar situation at the Sunrise Clinic, where Sr. Radebe reported high attrition rates from the Nutrition Therapeutic Program. The officials I interviewed attributed the attrition rate to women not wanting to queue for an additional service. In attempts to alleviate the long wait times, officials had suggested that facilities place the nutritional supplementation distribution as close to the antenatal clinic as possible. Sr. Radebe had other thoughts about why patients were not returning. "There's a stigma about getting food from the clinic," he said, "which causes people to default from the program."[7] He also mentioned a citywide stock shortage in March through August 2014. Patients who had attended had not received supplementation for those months and then had not returned to the clinic.

> The clients will come in and we have to tell them no, we don't have. They will come and sit in the waiting room and then they must wait until they get their folder and then when their folder is in my room, that's when they find out—after two hours or three hours—that's when they find out that the stock is not here. Sometimes the child loses weight, but we have to keep the child on the program because we don't know when the milk is going to come to the clinic. So we just keep them on the program and explain that we are running out of stock and we are still waiting for the stock. Sometimes this causes interruption.

Because those patients had not completed the program, they could not be coded as "successful" or "unsuccessful" and could only be coded as "interrupter/ defaulter." "Defaulters" could not be reentered into the program without a dietician's assessment, which presented a troubling situation: patients were penalized for their "failure" to complete a program that was dysfunctional. I asked one of the nurses about this problem, but he was at a loss as to how to answer me. "We recommend that the mother should be compliant," he said. When I asked what he meant by that, he explained that mothers should come to the clinic every month to check if the stock is available instead of interrupting the program.

Even when stock was available, the staff all noted that they repeatedly ran out of nutrition supplements before the end of the month, along with gloves and toilet paper. Dr. Lakay noted that for many patients the supplements constituted their family's main food source. "Supplements are not really supplements because it's the only food that some households have," she said. "You can get away without gloves, but a tin of milk? I don't have a substitute for that." She complained that the clinic focused on what was deemed "therapeutic" and ignored "preventive things like nutrition." Keeping the pharmacy well stocked with antiretrovirals was important, she said, but the nutrition supplements were also indispensable: "I mean, you must never say something like 'undernourishment causes AIDS' because then you'll start sounding like Thabo Mbeki, but you know, if you're run down, and not eating . . ." Dr. Lakay's reference to the Mbeki administration's insistence that it was inadequate nutrition, not HIV, that caused AIDS explained her hesitation about making the argument that a functioning Nutrition Therapeutic Program was as important as having enough antiretroviral medication. This tension is emblematic of the entangled history and persistent complexities of HIV and nutrition in South Africa (Cousins 2015). The example of the Nutrition Therapeutic Program shows that in the context of an already charged historical discourse around adherence to antiretroviral therapy (Robins 2006), patient responsibility was extended to adherence to pharmaceuticalized food, even in the face of systemic failures.

When Categories Do Not Hold

In addition to fundamental problems of infrastructure, lack of stock, broken or missing equipment, and procurement and storage issues, my interviews with clinic staff revealed other difficulties they encountered with the Nutrition Therapeutic Program protocol. Inevitably, there were instances when patients were not easily categorized. Sr. Yolwa spoke about how sometimes a child's MUAC and weight-for-height measurements would not correspond—one or the other would fall into the "normal" category, which then made it difficult to decide whether to refer the child to the Nutrition Therapeutic Program. "Then one must make a decision," she told me. Other staff agreed that in such instances they had to use their discretion and that it was wiser to refer the patient than to miss a potential case of undernutrition. "Sometimes you find that the MUAC is okay," Sr. Radebe told me, "and then you find that the weight is very low. Some of them they are so tricky, because you find out, their height for weight is okay, their MUAC is okay, but the weight, they keep on losing and going down. So that's when you have to decide—do I refer this child?"

Sr. Mbele added that measuring the weight, height, and MUAC and charting that data was not always enough. "The socioeconomic factors around Khayelitsha—some of them are not disclosing their info," he sighed. "But you will see when a person is poor—the appearance of the mom; the baby is dirty. So we check if there is a protruding stomach and we observe if there is edema in the feet. If both feet are swollen—that is one of the critical points of malnutrition." Sr. Mbele said that he referred about three children per week to the Nutrition Therapeutic Program, but he was concerned that cases were being missed. His seniors had also raised that concern after provincial audits of referrals. He attributed this to parents lying about exclusive breastfeeding or what they were feeding their children and to staff spending too much time excluding other causes of weight loss such as illness and focusing on certain signs and not others. He explained that the new protocol stipulated that all infants should be followed up at the clinic every month up to one year of age to prevent children being missed between immunization visits that were sometimes months apart. Staff had also been reminded to look for additional signs of malnutrition. "If you see that the hygiene is poor, or there's a skin problem, or the face of the baby is funny, that baby must be referred in. Because the baby might have a normal weight and mid-upper arm in some instances but when you check those signs, he has very long arms and a big stomach."

Sr. Mbele referred to these children as having severe malnutrition. Khayelitsha residents used the medical vernacular to describe such a child: a "kwash" baby—a colloquial shortening of kwashiorkor. During one discussion, Songezwa explained that the clinic requested that children were brought frequently for follow-up "because they don't want the babies to be kwash." I asked her what she meant by that. "When you see a baby with dry skin, underweight, big tummy, and big head and always the nose is running. It's more common in Ethiopia and Somalia—I have seen it on TV. But it is also common in the Eastern Cape and here in informal settlements." Like Sr. Mbele, Songezwa linked "kwash" to poor social circumstances: "It is common especially in those children of parents who drink a lot. Maybe they go to a shebeen for the whole weekend, and maybe they only feed the child on Thursday night and then leftovers on Sunday. In my area we have a neighbor like that. There were seven children in that house and the social worker has taken five of them already."

As Sr. Mbele pointed out, the "kwash" baby can confound protocol. Weight and length and MUAC measurements and the mandatory check for pedal edema as

per Integrated Management of Childhood Illness guidelines might be insufficient to detect severe malnutrition. To err on the side of caution is to allow for
the subjective assessment of the health care professional, who might notice
changes in hair, dry skin, or a "funny face"—details that are less easily captured
and ticked off on a protocol. It is an instance in which intuition must override
the "instrumental rationality" (Good 1994) of clinical medicine, the tendency to
focus on instrumental knowledge as the basis for rational decision-making.

The increasing number of children classified as overweight or obese posed a
different challenge to clinic staff. One of the pediatric nurses said to me one
morning: "Yesterday I saw a child who missed his last date and now he is overweight. Now what must I do?" I reminded her that I was not employed by the
clinic, but we agreed that this was a good question. What is the protocol for
the follow-up or management of overweight children? A senior nurse clarified
later that these children should be referred to the dietician. In the context of a
roaming dietician who visited the clinic only once a month, this seemed like
a piecemeal solution.

Staff were also unsure about what to do with patients who might be categorized as "food insecure." Dr. Mokoena, assuming I had some knowledge about
the nutritional services at the clinic, asked me one morning to explain how the
clinic's referral system to local food projects worked. She showed me the form
that had been dispensed to staff some months earlier: "Referral for Nutritional
Assistance at Local Feeding Site/Food Security Pilot Project." The form said:
"This patient, who does not meet the inclusion criteria for the Nutrition Therapeutic Program of the Health Facility-Based Nutrition Program, is food insecure. It would be appreciated if you could supply the patient or household with
the necessary food support. Thank you." Dr. Mokoena was not sure where to
send patients after filling out this form. "I don't know where to send them, so
obviously the patient gets lost," she fretted. I was not aware of any external feeding schemes and suggested that we ask the clinic manager. The manager con-
firmed that the clinic no longer had an external feeding referral site and there was
no alternative for food insecure patients who did not meet the inclusion criteria
for the Nutrition Therapeutic Program. I relayed this back to Dr. Mokoena, who
had completed the form a few times and kept it in patients' folders. Nutrition
protocols overlooked and did not make provision for food insecurity as a factor
that shaped the clinical nutrition profiles of women and children despite the
high prevalence of food insecurity in this group.

When I asked staff during interviews who was in charge of the Nutrition Therapeutic Program, their answers differed. Some thought that it was Sr. Qoma's job
(she took care of stock), while others sent patients to Sr. Radebe. Sr. Radebe told
me that "everyone" was doing Nutrition Therapeutic Program work. He had
taken on Sr. Yolwa's extra caseload during her maternity leave and could not do all
the Nutrition Therapeutic Program referrals himself. The administration of the

Nutrition Therapeutic Program at the Sunrise and Kunye clinics thus corresponded with an evaluation of the program in the Western Cape that concluded that a "lack of strategic organization and no clear responsibility for distribution at clinic level must be suspected of causing obstacles to efficiency and program coverage" (Hansen et al. 2015, 4). This evaluation also found that the program was not subject to internal assessment at clinics, which meant that such problems were not detected. At the Sunrise Clinic, although auditing was a prominent feature of managers' and clinicians' workloads, the Nutrition Therapeutic Program was somehow overlooked.

The Audit

It was Dr. Foster's job to audit clinical folders as part of the Sunrise Clinic's quality of care evaluation. "The audit looks at a variety of things," he explained, "like organization of the folders, completion of the folder, record keeping, history taking, explaining investigations, physical examination, diagnosis, management of the patient, and health education." He showed me the preformatted audit tool and the clinic stationery that should be used by staff. "It is a well-designed form, a nice little summary of the patient. And then because it is all outlined, you don't have to write much down, you just tick and classify. And then over the back, you've got room for their plan." He took a folder to demonstrate how he would go about auditing it. "I start off with completion of the folder. The sticker scores most of that. And then the only other thing you're looking for is whether they took next-of-kin detail and a phone number, which almost never happens. Then you go to"—he opened the folder to look for the standard form—"this one doesn't have one; it just has a note. So already I know that this one is going to score badly—they have just done a more traditional sort of format. It is not to say that this isn't a decent consult, and this patient is neglected, but because they haven't written down that they've checked a lot of things, it will score badly. So I've tried educating the sisters about that concept: that if you don't write it down, it didn't happen."

The audit tool included a section with the heading "Malnutrition/Anemia." I asked Dr. Foster what would be expected of the nurse for this section. His response illustrates some of the problems of an overly protocol-based approach to care and a lack of a backup when such protocols fail:

> It's pretty simple stuff. They're just looking to plot the weight and see if it is tracking well and if it is normal. And for anemia, it's really just whether they are pale or not. So it's really a gross evaluation. But that's one of the things where I've tried to, you know, educate that if that kid is not growing well, you should test the hemoglobin. Don't just go on pallor. If you're concerned about nutrition you need to check. So this is only really designed as a screening tool and in most cases, it results in appropriate treatment of the child, but it often misses things. There's not really

anything on development in here, which would probably take too long to do in an assessment, but if the child is not growing properly [according to the Road to Health booklet], then automatically you are supposed to do a feeding assessment. So the form works well as a screen. In terms of getting them referred to the right place, the form lets us down I think because if they have any other danger signs, they are supposed to immediately refer to the doctor. Whereas if they have got poor growth there's nothing that says they have to immediately refer, which I think is a big miss. Because I see a lot of that in my audits: that the kid has been growing poorly for months now, and they have done a feeding assessment but then there is no real plan, we've just identified that the kid's got malnutrition or that something else is going on. But then there's no appropriate plan and follow-up made.

Children flagged as "sick" based on the protocol's listed "danger signs," such as respiratory problems, fever, and/or diarrhea, would be referred to the doctor. Children flagged as "malnourished" based on their growth parameters were not referred to the doctor because the protocol stipulated that they be referred to Nutrition Therapeutic Program and then to the dietician if that failed. Dr. Foster said that he was not involved in the Nutrition Therapeutic Program and that the "immunization and HIV sisters" were in charge of that program. In sum, the clinical audit tended to overlook nutrition. If it is filled out properly, the Road to Health Booklet may have provided information about child growth, but often these records are not fully completed (Manderson and Ross 2020).

As Dr. Foster described these problems to me, he defended his colleagues as having done their best despite resource constraints, and he did not equate the audit scores with quality of care:

The problem is if you score badly on this it doesn't necessarily mean that you haven't taken good care of the patient. These are just certain things that management have decided they want done. If there is a bad score, I'm not necessarily fussed with the way the patient was managed because it might be little things that lowered the score. The sisters are not being deliberately neglectful; it's because they're not trained to recognize certain things. I mean you can't replace a doctor. Basically. And they do the best they can. But it is a useful tool in that it helps me to identify common problems in the management of children, and then I can address these. I usually go to the individual sisters because it is less confrontational. But I have spoken to all of them a few times on certain things, like signing of notes, writing your name and designation, and more general things that you can apply to adults and children.

Dr. Foster engaged in what Hannah Brown (2016) has termed "empathetic bureaucracy," which acknowledges that management is not just about tools and techniques but also about social relations, such that it consists of both governance and care. Given the practices of audit and evaluation that policy implementation demands, staff must navigate between these modalities of the technical and the relational.

LIFE BETWEEN PROTOCOLS

Staff accounts of the nutrition and lifestyle education package that is part of their clinical mandate revealed incongruences between what they knew should be said as part of health education and what they felt could be done by patients given their circumstances. The rote dispensing of advice might be one example of what Guillaume Lachenal (2015, 107) has labeled "medical nihilism": a renouncing of action given that "nothing can be done." However, my observations in the clinic pointed to a web of care relations that did not fit into clinical flow diagrams. Health care workers' negotiations of stock shortages, high patient loads, missing folders, lack of stationery, and failing infrastructure reflected a logic of care (Mol 2008) that navigated around and through standardized frameworks.

On the other side of the consulting desk, patients' experiences of the perinatal nutrition policy illustrated the tendency of life to fall outside protocol perimeters. The hard reality of hunger in Khayelitsha, where a "normal" or "overweight" body mass index does not mean that a patient is food secure, was a far cry from the abstractions of the clinical approach to antenatal nutrition based on MUAC measurements, micronutrients, and ready-to-use therapeutic food. But a discussion of life between protocols must begin where it is most directly embodied: in the waiting room.

Waiting

A visit to the clinic is a whole-day affair. Patients who want to be seen first arrive an hour before the 8 A.M. opening time, and even then they are likely to be at the clinic for four hours or more. Although staff have tried to improve the system, patient flow is slow and involves multiple stops (reception, observations room, consulting room, pharmacy), each of which has its own waiting time. Most of a patient's time in the clinic will be spent in waiting areas as they move from one room to the next. Table 2 illustrates Inam's visit to the clinic one month after delivery and offers a typical snapshot.

"It's unfortunate in the public service that patients have to wait," Dr. Foster told me. "You really are going to wait a long time." Dr. Mokoena said that "patients can be difficult. There is a sense of entitlement. They want to be seen and they want to be seen now." Dr. Foster agreed that patients' expectations were problematic. "It just never seems to sink in [that you have to wait]. Patients often jump the queue and they come straight to a sister or a doctor, despite being told repeatedly that that is not appropriate," he said. "It's a problem, just trying to

TABLE 2 Inam's day at the clinic

7:45 a.m.	Arrive at clinic
8:00 a.m.	Clinic doors open. Inam hands in the baby's clinic card at reception so they can retrieve her folder. Inam is offered a surgical mask on arrival but refuses to wear it.
8:15 a.m.	Waiting in reception area.
9:08 a.m.	Inam is called and is asked to retrieve her own folder from the clerks because she needs another HIV test as per PMTCT protocol. She sits down again.
9:25 a.m.	The clerk calls out the names of patients whose folders have been retrieved, but not Inam's name.
9:30 a.m.	The clerk suggests that Inam weigh the baby while they retrieve the folders and Inam goes to a second waiting area, the one for the observations room.
9:34 a.m.	The clerk returns and reports that her folder and the baby's folder cannot be found. The clerk directs Inam to the help desk to fill in a form to create two new folders.
9:40 a.m.	Inam returns to the observations waiting area.
9:45 a.m.	Inam is called to the observations room so the baby can be weighed. Inam undresses the baby on the counter. The sister weighs the baby and records the weight on Inam's hand: 3.6 kilograms.
9:47 a.m.	Inam dresses the baby in the changing room and returns to the reception waiting area to wait for new folders.
10:32 a.m.	The baby's folder arrives; Inam's is not yet available. She is asked to wait.
10:51 a.m.	Inam's old folder is found in the observations room. She is directed to HIV counseling for an HIV test.
11:03 a.m.	Inam returns and we move back to the observations waiting area.
11:07 a.m.	Inam is called into the observations room. The nurse records observations in the folder.
11:14 a.m.	Inam moves to the consultations waiting area.
12:55 p.m.	Inam is called into the consultation room for baby's one-month checkup.
1:00 p.m.	The consultation is finished and Inam is given a follow-up appointment in six weeks.
1:05 p.m.	Inam hands in her folder at reception and we leave the clinic.

explain to patients that they're not more special than other patients. Because their reasoning is that they shouldn't have to wait and other patients should. That's something I've tried to change with an appointment system and that's improved things but not fixed things."

Inam's clinic visit for a routine follow-up one month after delivery took five hours and twenty minutes. Of that time, she spent approximately twenty minutes with different health care professionals and approximately five hours waiting in different parts of the clinic. Among my participants, this would be considered a good day, given that Inam was out by lunchtime. Some patients had sat in the clinic until closing time only to be told to return the next day. For example, at one of her visits Nobomi was asked to return to the clinic for test results a week after her blood was taken. At her return visit, the nurse had difficulty accessing the laboratory results but asked Nobomi to wait as she had hoped to get through to the laboratory by the end of the day. She could not access the results in the end and Nobomi left the clinic after an eight-hour wait with the advice that she should return in the morning. It is unclear why the nurse did not offer to phone her with the results when she learned that the system was offline. In general, patients usually spent between four and eight hours in the clinic for their appointments with one exception: grant day.

On grant day, the queue in the waiting room was displaced to queues that snaked out of banks, supermarkets, and halls across Khayelitsha. "People are elsewhere sorting out their financials," Sr. Mbele explained to me. Grant days are the first two working days of the month. Each person who receives a grant (a child welfare grant, pension, or disability grant) takes their South African Social Security Agency (SASSA) card to draw their monthly funds from a cash machine if they have a chipped card or to swipe the card at a participating supermarket to pay for groceries or to draw the cash at the till (the Shoprite, Spar, and Pick n Pay supermarkets participate in this scheme). "On grant day, they separate the tills," Nomsa explained, "some are SASSA only. The money must be withdrawn by the seventh day of the month. If it is not, they might not give you the money. They will see that you are not desperate." When they were not queuing for health care, people were queuing for welfare payments or food, or both.

Waiting is central to the patient's experience of public sector health care in South Africa. While for the most part not much activity takes place while patients sit and wait, there are some distractions. Health promotion talks take place a few times a week, the oral rehydration station is purposefully kept in the waiting area for quick attention to dehydrated children, and the scale stands in the waiting area so that patients can be weighed while they wait. The waiting area is frequently so full that patients stand against the windows or convert the clinic's trashcans into makeshift stools. Some of the blue plastic seating is cracked and mothers roll up their baby blankets to cushion the seats. People chat, toddlers gurgle, and there is the sporadic rustle of a chip packet. Some people have smartphones for entertainment; others close their eyes and try to nap. Children pace and bounce between the aisles of plastic chairs.

Unsurprisingly, the mood in the waiting room was one of fatigue and boredom. Yet the waiting room was also a microcosm that revealed the endurance and care that characterized mothers' dispositions in everyday life. As caregivers sat waiting, their time was punctuated by entertaining, comforting, or feeding their children. They bought lollipops for 50 cents at the clinic entrance—the universal treat that comes with a trip to the clinic, a gift, a panacea for the boredom, and a therapeutic adjunct, like the kiss on the forehead that makes the child well again. Waiting, in this frame, becomes an act of love, a suspension between the now of the child who demands constant attention and presence and the later, the potential that is promised—if only one will wait.

Therapeutic Nutrition?

On paper, the antenatal nutrition protocol is straightforward: based on BMI and MUAC measurements, women are either categorized as "undernourished," in which case they qualify for nutritional supplementation, or they are categorized as "normal" or "overweight," in which case they should receive counseling about "nutrition and lifestyle." As the cases of Inam and Sindi show, these classifications fail to address social questions about food security and hunger.

Inam was started on the Nutrition Therapeutic Program after being classified as underweight. As we sat together in her small kitchen, Inam shrugged and told me that she had always been thin. Trained as a journalist, she was working for a media company in central Cape Town when she became pregnant, and her work schedule meant that she often skipped meals. She also described herself as "fussy" about food. She had adopted a vegan lifestyle some years ago but was reluctantly incorporating more animal protein into her diet now that she was pregnant again. She opened one of the kitchen cupboards to show me the cereals, milkshakes, and sachets of peanut butter she had received. The packaging for the porridge she had been given stated that "apart from the direct benefits [of this product] on the immune system, long-term benefits regarding prevention of degenerative diseases of lifestyle are a distinct possibility." The peanut butter was labeled as a "ready-to-use food supplement, RUTF F-100 formula." These products are made by a Cape Town–based company whose slogan is "manufacturers of food for wellness." According to its webpage, the company aims to serve both South Africa's nutraceutical market and "nutrition crisis zones around the world." Inam followed the nurses' advice to use the food supplements despite her dislike for them. "You can taste the medication in there," she grimaced. The milkshakes and porridge were manageable, but not the peanut butter, which she described as too sweet. Inam took the peanut butter sachets from the clinic anyway: they would always be consumed by someone in her large household. The children would frequently eat the porridge, milk, and peanut butter that Inam received from the clinic. As the breadwinner for a household of seven, Inam was food secure, unlike many of the other women I met, who were categorized as "overweight" at the clinic and who were not eligible for food supplements but who experienced frequent hunger. Nevertheless, Inam was unhappy when the supplements were stopped postnatally because she was concerned about weight loss from breastfeeding. "After the baby's born, they don't give it to you anymore," she said.

I met Sindi on only one occasion, in the waiting room. But the long wait meant that we had many hours to discuss how she was faring with her pregnancy and her thoughts on the clinic's interventions. Sindi was categorized as "normal" weight and received nutrition and lifestyle counseling during her first antenatal visit as well as pamphlets to take home. She told me about her frustrations with the dietary information the clinic dispensed. "I know what a healthy diet looks like," she said. "It's just a matter of money. If I had money I would eat and do whatever I want to do. I know my diet is not good enough, so I take a supplement—Centrum Maternal." She was aware of the advice to follow a certain diet and to exercise but explained that "these things are there, we see them, but we can't really do them. It's not really accessible." Her food choices—where she shopped and what she bought—were financial choices. She went to Shoprite rather than the rival chain Pick n Pay because it was cheaper, albeit a bit "untidy." She shopped in Khayelitsha because transporting groceries from farther away was difficult even though she was aware that in the township "some foods are not really accessible." Sindi said that if she had more money, she would buy food from outside Khayelitsha, including goods not on offer in the township, such as fresh fish and strawberries. "If I had money, I would limit my food intake and eat smaller portions. I'd eat a different diet every day, rather than the same rice, pap [maize porridge], cabbage. I know I eat too much carbohydrate—rice, potato, butternut, cabbage, carrots, samp [crushed corn], and beans, not the fancy food that you see on TV." Like many of my participants, Sindi emphasized that following nutritional advice—having smaller portions, eating a variety of foods, and focusing on fruit and vegetables—was possible only for the financially secure. For everyone else, there was little option but to buy cheaper food that kept you feeling full. As Songezwa put it, "You can't be full with only vegetables, but in the clinic they don't mention pap or rice or samp and beans. Vegetables, chicken liver, fish, meat, milk, and yoghurt, but no pap or rice or samp and beans, even though we know that they [the nursing staff] eat that as well!"

For some, the clinic's failure to provide a meal during the antenatal visit, especially after giving birth, was an affront. Lindiwe compared her experience at the local midwife obstetric unit with a friend who had delivered at a private hospital: "A friend of mine gave birth at Melomed [a private clinic] and afterwards her boyfriend took a photo of her with this nice meal. The local clinic, they don't give any meal." At the midwife obstetric unit, women are discharged six hours after uncomplicated deliveries and receive tea and a slice of bread or biscuits during that time. Aviwe recounted how a local NGO provided meals for pregnant women waiting for antenatal care at a clinic she attended during her first pregnancy:

At that place they cook for the pregnant patients. They ask you, "Did you eat?" If you didn't eat, they take you to the side to eat something and they say "Come back after you have eaten." They don't even ask here—they just give the injection. They say "Sisi, I'm going to give an injection because you have a discharge. I'm going to give you these pills." I said okay. But I know it is not right. Because what if I didn't even have a banana in my stomach? Maybe you feel dizzy, you feel hungry, you see? Sometimes some of us don't have something to eat. . . . Some of us don't even have partners now. Some partners left when they were two months, three months pregnant, you see? And this person is not working, she is struggling, you see man, they are supposed to give food for people that go there. They can't just . . . they didn't even ask me before they injected me.

FOOD, SUPPLEMENTS, AND PHARMACEUTICALS: CITIZENS, PATIENTS, AND CLIENTS

My participants' perspectives on the Nutrition Therapeutic Program and nutrition counseling and their concern that the clinic did not provide meals illustrate two tensions. The first is the blurring of food and pharmaceuticals in perinatal policy. Cooked food offered during waiting time, peanut butter in sterile sachets, and over-the-counter vitamin supplements are substances that connote "food" or "pharmaceutical" in different measures. While the clinic was able to provide supplements for those who met the inclusion criteria, it did not provide food.

Aligned with the categories "food", "pharmaceutical", and the hybrid "food supplement" are the shifting categories of "citizen", "patient", and "client". There is a constant negotiation of the uncertain boundaries between the affirmation of rights-based access to state provisions and calls for the rights-bearing subject to care for herself. In the context of a policy focus on the first 1,000 days, this logic extends to include care for a future individual, configured as both a citizen endowed with future human capital and a patient or client whose future biological risk is attenuated by prescriptions of ready-to-use-therapeutic food. In this context, ready-to-use foods are not emergency provisions as part of a humanitarian intervention, as they have been described elsewhere (Redfield 2012; Scott-Smith 2013; Stellmach 2016). In the same way that Donna Haraway (1997) has argued that agribusiness technologies and computers in financial capitals are as much reproductive technologies as sonograms and IVF, RUTFs in this context are reproductive technologies meant to secure the future (Pentecost and Cousins 2018).

Just as antiretroviral provisioning in southern Africa has revealed a chronic hunger that unsettles notions of adherence (Kalofonos 2010; Cousins 2016), the Nutrition Therapeutic Program and the nutrition and lifestyle education of pregnant women reveals contradictory logics of rights and responsibilities. The perinatal nutrition policy and its placing of patients into two broad categories— those who receive assistance in the form of food supplementation and those who are called on to make responsible choices and self-make as citizens— reflects the new "politics of distribution" in South Africa (Ferguson 2015). Inclusion and exclusion from a stake in state resources hinges on more than citizenship or its therapeutic variants (Nguyen 2010). It is also predicated on forms of intimacy seen as worthy (Berlant 1998; Povinelli 2006)—in this case, the mother-child dyad—and on a normative notion of agency whose opposite is irresponsibility, noncompliance, incapability, or intransigence (Berlant 2007).

Yet the accounts of pregnant women reveal a second tension, between the focus of nutrition policy on the individual and the inadequacies of that policy for attending to the structural problems of food insecurity and food availability. As the stories of Sindi, Lindiwe, and Aviwe show, food "choices" in Khayelitsha reflect a political economy characterized by the globalization of cheap food and the provision of therapeutic food to a select few via state, philanthropic, and market networks, based on an entangled logic of state mandates, humanitarianism, and entrepreneurialism (Pentecost and Cousins 2018). This contrasts starkly with the human rights discourse of "the right to have access to sufficient food and water" enshrined in Section 27(1)(b) of the Constitution of the Republic of South Africa and the constitutional mandate for the state to "take reasonable legislative and other measures, within its available resources, to achieve the progressive realization of each of these rights." As Maggie Dickinson (2019) has documented in the United States and Alyshia Gálvez (2018) in Mexico, the privileging of market logics over social welfare produces a food system that does little to secure the right to food while also manifesting new burdens of metabolic disease and directing responsibility away from the state and toward individuals.

Access to nutritious food, particularly during pregnancy and early life, is the fundamental issue underlying a focus on the first 1,000 days. This access is not secured via a constitutional mandate but is rather subject to the second tenet of the politics of potential: that responsibility for manifesting potential lies with the individual. The contradictions at play here are evident to women who are the subject of these policies and to clinic staff. They were well aware of the challenges their patients described and dealt with them in a manner that shifted between engagement and care, fatigue and nihilism.

Bracketing Advice

The range of attitudes among staff members toward the lifestyle education package might be described as on a spectrum from nihilism to care. Health care workers were acutely aware of what Sr. Mbele referred to as "the socioeconomic factors in Khayelitsha" and dealt with this disjuncture in several ways. Many framed socioeconomic problems as beyond the remit of the clinic. Others offered well-meaning but unrealistic suggestions for ways that patients might adhere to the health and nutrition advice. While it was clear that many staff members were resigned about the boundaries of their abilities to deal with the significant challenges faced by their patients, it was also apparent that many of them were dedicated to offering care.

Almost every staff member interviewed expressed reservations about whether patients could easily follow the nutrition and health advice they received at the clinic given the constraints in the community. Sr. Radebe threw up his hands during our interview. "The environment is not therapeutic," he told me. "We are seeing diarrhea in children because of water dumped in front of their houses. And the dirt—there's no vehicle picking up the bins. Lack of sanitation. Maybe five houses using one toilet. Father is not working, mother is not working. There are programs that give out food parcels but that doesn't happen often. And that does not alleviate the poverty in the house."

Sr. Josephs similarly framed the issues that hindered patients from following nutrition and lifestyle advice as related to "poverty"—a word that, as Akhil Gupta (2012, 22) has argued, obscures violence to make its bureaucratic management "unexceptional, a matter of routine administration". As was the case in many of my conversations with clinic staff, Sr. Josephs cited these issues as falling under the jurisdiction of social workers:

I don't know how to put it. . . . Financially, most people don't work so they can't afford to buy things, you see. Vegetables for them are like so . . . they think they are so pricey. But ja, they do get grants some of them, somehow, but they cannot buy groceries that will be nutritionally good for them. It's a very poor area socially, most people are not working and they're staying in shacks and they share. You find that it is a family of six, sharing one shack and she has to feed all these children and she's not working. She's getting grants for two babies maybe— that is now the social grant that they get here in South Africa, it's 300 rand[8] or something, you know—so she must now buy groceries and you can see that she will not be able to feed herself and take care of the baby that she is pregnant with if she has to feed that whole family. It goes way back, because people in this area, they are financially deprived, their way of living is not that good, they are poverty-stricken, I must say, I must say it like that . . . you see, so it is quite, it's quite difficult to actually come up with a . . . I don't know . . . that will help these clients. You have to look into all those aspects. And to be honest, we have nothing here. No facility that helps them regarding that, but we advise them to see social workers, who can actually attend to them and help them, because social workers will go to their households and see what is going on and see how they can assist them.

Dr. Mokoena expressed empathy for patients' circumstances but was similarly resigned about the boundaries of her role in addressing these:

It is really, really difficult to say to someone who is very obese or overweight "Eat healthy," because that entails having vegetables and having money to buy all the healthy things, whereas the little money they do have is to buy your basic grains— your mielie [maize] meal, your samp, your porridge, and your oil, and that's what they live on because it is sustainable and it is what they can afford, so ja, when we educate we are always going on about healthy diet healthy diet healthy diet, but in the back of our minds we know that it is difficult. Even though I advise them to have more vegetables and more fruit, some of them will say to me: "But doctor where must I get money for that? The money I have is only my grant money and that's enough for my 2.5 kilos of mielie meal and samp." And I hear what they are saying. I am not in their shoes. All I can do is advise them, tell them the risks of what they are eating, you know, but at the end of the day honestly there's really nothing I can do for them.

Some staff explained that they tried to shape advice with the client's circumstances in mind. Staff acknowledged the difficulties of preparing healthy food for a large family when everyone in the house "eats from the same pot" and family members might not agree about new cooking methods or adding more vegetables. They advised buying inexpensive food items that were designated as "healthy" in the nutrition protocols, such as lentils, or making small changes such as adding less salt to food, and many referred to food gardens as a way for clients to increase their intake of healthy food. This was the case in my interview with Sr. Mbuli:

SM: We always encourage the free stuff like vegetables, fruits, water . . .
MP: When you say "the free stuff"—is it available? Fruit and vegetables?
SM: No, but if they can plant fruit in their houses, it will be free after that . . .
MP: Right. Do you think that's quite common, that people plant things in the garden?
SM: There are, there are . . . but very few.

Mrs. Tshabalala echoed this idea:

MT: Sometimes when you tell them "you must eat this and that," they will ask "where are we going to get that?" So we introduce to them the veggies, the garden. Maybe they don't have the space, you know. Maybe they are living in a squatter camp and their shack is behind the others. So then maybe it is a container garden. So for them, it's . . .
MP: It is very difficult to garden?
MT: It's very difficult, but there are those who are making the container garden.

Dr. Mokoena also thought this was a good idea but that it needed to be a broader community project:

If you say to someone, "Have your own vegetable garden"—where? You know, they are living on top of each other, where are they going to grow these vegetables? I remember some communities have vegetable gardens that they do as a combined effort for that particular community. I've seen one on Spine Road.[9]

There is a little garden there. It's quite small, it won't feed the whole of Khayelitsha, but it is probably a food project that someone started. I think maybe that in townships each block should have a little food garden and maybe you share whatever comes out of that. Because there is no space, people don't have space, because they live in shacks.

Sr. Radebe was less enthusiastic about community food security programs. "There are programs that give people food parcels or set up gardens, but that doesn't happen often." This aligned more closely with research findings on food security in Khayelitsha, which have shown that small-scale urban agriculture is rarely practiced and does not significantly contribute to food security (Battersby 2011). I spent a day in the waiting room talking to Zekiswa, a young woman who was attending for family planning and who lived in one of the most deprived parts of Khayelitsha. She expressed a similar sentiment about the short-lived community development projects in her area: "I'm telling you—after a week, you'll no longer find that new project, there's no money in it, and those people who came with that project, they will eat the money."

Other staff members simply advised their clients to "work with what was at home." Sr. Yeka explained this to me using the example of a child who is not gaining weight:

It is not that they [mothers] don't want to cook or what, they just don't have the stuff to cook for the children. I advise to cook porridge in the morning. If they have margarine or a teaspoon of cooking oil, they can add five milliliters a day for the child. Now we have peanut butter for the nutrition [program] so they could use peanut butter if they have . . . or the sort of thing they have at home. You have to turn it into the food for the child. I try to advise them—whatever you have at home, just turn it into a food for a child.

Staff were at a loss about how to approach the difficulties of offering nutritional advice with the knowledge that this advice was incongruent with the daily realities of life in Khayelitsha. There was a hollow note to their statements that reflect not a lack of concern but rather desperation—the desire to offer something instead of nothing. The challenges of clinical work in this setting should not be underestimated. The high patient volume, the frequent lack of equipment and stock, staff shortages, the difficulty of obtaining lab results, the inefficiencies of patient flow, and the loss of patient folders (and thus clinical records) were common problems. The impact on service provision, as staff explained to me, was significant and often at the expense of clinical time with the patient. Although staff were sympathetic about the difficulties their patients faced, they confined their engagement to a narrow clinical mandate that tended to route responsibility back to the individual because of the constraints of the clinic. As Sr. Qoma put it, "I can only do what I can, and all I can do is just explain to the client." Such a statement encapsulates a kind of medical nihilism that at worst is an apathy and disregard at odds with the values the health profession espouses and at best is a reflection of the fatigue and burnout that characterizes health care workers' experiences of the public sector. I suggest the latter, given that I also observed many instances when staff members extended care.

The Pragmatics of Care

Despite the feelings of helplessness and frustration staff described, more often than not I observed that they were deeply invested in offering care. They navigated protocols and recommendations to bring the maximum benefit to patients, they frequently worked after hours to ensure that all the patients were attended to, and they actively engaged with issues such as the flow of patients between different sections, even trialing an alternative triage system during my time there to decrease waiting times.

Sr. Mbele, among others, worked late if there were more children to be seen because he feared that if he sent them away, they would not return. "We see more than four hundred patients a day. And you feel like, 'I'm not doing [this] properly.' You are looking at the time." Sr. Mbele shook his head. "It is not supposed to be like that."

Staff would err on the side of referring clients to the nutrition therapeutic program. Sr. Qoma, distressed by the nutritional supplement stock shortages and concerned that patients would "interrupt" the program, did not request, as some other nurses did, that patients come back once a month to check if the stock had arrived so she could tick off their attendance. She gave her mobile number to her patients so they could send her a text message to see if the stock had arrived before making the trip to the clinic. During the stock shortage, she also began to ration the supplements so that all the patients on the program would get something. While this was far from ideal in terms of the protocol, it was more pragmatic to offer each client half the usual supplement package than it was to stick firmly to the rules and thus provide supplements to fewer patients. Sr. Qoma was also diligent about contacting patients who had not returned. After a skipped visit she would phone them, and if that failed, she would ensure that a community health worker went to the home address the patient had given to investigate why they had not attended.

Sr. Qoma navigated the change in the infant feeding policy by continuing to give formula to HIV-positive women who requested it for as long as possible. "I just give [formula]. As long as the government is giving out and I can still order those two hundred tins a month, why not give?" she told me. "I'll keep doing that until there is something written down." At the same time, she was discerning about when to follow the existing written directive (give women a choice) and when to follow the tentative recommendations of managers to promote exclusive breastfeeding pending the formal policy notice. If a patient was working, for example, Sr. Qoma would tell her that she could not provide formula, reasoning that employed women could buy their own. In this way, she allocated clinic resources to the patients she perceived as most needy through selective adoption of the new preliminary policy when it was useful.

For some of the staff members, care was bound up in a close affinity with the challenges their patients faced. While the nursing profession in South Africa enjoys a respectable authority and middle-class status, many practitioners share their patients' backgrounds and thus occupy contradictory social positions (Marks 1994). This may reinforce paternal and moralizing forms of care (Le Marcis and Girard 2015) or, as in the case of Sr. Lolo, accentuate empathy with patients' hardships. Sr. Lolo lived in another township nearby. She worked in the observations room and saw all of the children for their weight and height measurements. On the wall at her station, she kept a faded sepia photo of herself and her eldest son. She had two more children, but her second-born had died in his teens following a fatal stab wound. Sr. Lolo's empathy for young mothers was palpable: she had both a commanding presence that marshaled mothers and babes in the small space of the prep room and a soft demeanor that quickly consoled toddlers screaming at the prospect of having to sit on the scale.

Staff cared for each other as well. Nearly every staff member I interviewed mentioned the satisfaction they derived from working in a close-knit team. When Sr. Lolo turned 60 at the end of 2014, the clinic staff threw a party for her in the tearoom, complete with cake, soft drinks, and a large banner that read "Happy 60th Birthday!" The banner remained on the tearoom notice board, a happy reminder of the staff party. Parties for colleagues, daily morning meetings, and sharing tea together were some of the ways clinic workers supported each other. The nurses all wore their crisp, white, formal uniforms on Spring Day—a "morale booster," as Sr. Qoma put it. The doctors often took their tea breaks together, which provided not only a respite but also a chance to help each other with clinical difficulties. In this way, health care workers endured the inherent contradictions of work that connotes the alleviation of suffering, but in actuality must "unknow" suffering that cannot be alleviated by means of a protocol (Geissler 2013; Pentecost 2018a).

NIHILISM AND CARE

In this chapter, I have considered the particularities of biomedical practice that characterize contemporary African global health and have shown that this practice is always relational. While the ideas and practices that constitute the clinic extend beyond its physical borders, the material infrastructures that constitute clinical spaces should not be overlooked. The clinic—a contested image in fragile states elsewhere (Geissler 2015a)—still constitutes an important space of governmentality in the South African context. As Lauren Muller (2004, 54) has written in her work on the geography of the clinic in the Western Cape, local primary health care is constituted by "particular facilities and communities, places which are not merely sites of instrumental biomedical practice, but buildings, spaces and associated social relations with particular meanings and attachment for individuals and communities that use and occupy them."

Protocols and their sites of implementation have a "local universality" in that their "universality always rests on real-time work, and emerges from localized processes of negotiations and pre-existing institutional, infrastructural, and material relations" (Timmermans and Berg 1997, 275). In one sense, this seems self-evident. For policy to be enacted, actors must interpret it and use their discretion to best apply it in their contexts. Given that standardized protocols cannot make provision for all possible contingencies, health care work is necessarily characterized by a continuous negotiation of formal policy and clinical pragmatism (Timmermans and Almeling 2009). Dr. Foster's auditing work exemplifies this approach: he follows up with nursing staff when issues arise but is also willing to overlook deviations from the protocol if he is satisfied that the quality of care was adequate.

In another sense, though, there are subtler underpinnings of the uneven manner in which policy is practiced. Lives are evaluated differently, and in the case of perinatal policy, that evaluation rests on body mass indices, mid-upper arm circumference measurements, CD4 counts, and HIV viral loads. These metrics determine level of care, access to additional food supplementation, method of infant feeding, and the moral prescriptions that accompany nutrition education. The use of these metrics also variably configures women in the role of welfare recipients, self-making responsible citizens, and guardians of the future. This logic configures the distribution of resources and the disposition of institutions tasked with distributing them. In the context of the clinic, it allows for knowledge of what staff termed "socioeconomic factors" without acknowledgment of the reality of hunger this term obscures (see also Cousins 2016). It allows for the "unknowing" (Geissler 2013) of hunger, based on the fact that nothing can be done within the protocol.

In his work on HIV in Cameroon, Guillaume Lachenal (2015, 132) proposes nihilism as "a heuristic hypothesis to examine the place of hubris, simulation, and pretense in the politics and techniques of global health in Africa." Lachenal uses this heuristic to problematize a common narrative of public health in Africa that exaggerates the importance of novel biopolitical forms with the advent of globalized neoliberalism and declining nation-states. If we wish to examine how African biomedicine has changed in the era of global health, Lachenal suggests, we should look not only to the material effects that signal such changes but also to what is purposefully *not said* or *not done*. The action—or more often inaction—of health care workers in my observations can be understood as shaded with a medical nihilism, a renouncing of action given that "nothing can be done." In nearly all of my interactions, clinic staff resorted to platitudes such as "To be honest, we have nothing here." As Dr. Mokoena concluded: "At the end of the day honestly there's really nothing I can do for them."

And yet clinic staff must deliver nutritional advice as part of the clinical mandate. Producing registers and completing forms *represents* a functioning system. As Lachenal has noted for the era of global health, "spectacle, under this regime, is what matters" (2015, 133). It matters that there is a visible sign that warns of the potential threat of Ebola infection, a token of the global biosecurity complex at the entrance to this small clinic. *WASH YOUR HANDS OFTEN. Use SOAP. Do not touch an infected person.* It does not matter that residents of the informal settlement served by this clinic live in some of the most unsanitary conditions in the city and that raw sewage frequently flows past their yards. It matters that a register exists with a record of all the patients enrolled in the Nutrition Therapeutic Program. It does not matter that three-quarters of those patients have "defaulted." It matters that Dr. Mokoena has done the paperwork to refer her patient to a "local feeding site." It does not matter that such a facility no longer exists.

Drawing on Achille Mbembe's rendering of postcolonial state logics and aesthetics as obscene or even absurd (2001), Lachenal (2015, 108) "pictures global biomedicine in Africa not so much in terms of greed, extraction and surveillance, but rather as a world of inaction and impotence." While the constraints of clinical work in Khayelitsha are real, they are also often a justification for just ticking the boxes and overlooking the boxes that are not ticked. Encouraging patients to access "the free stuff" or suggesting that people living in tightly packed shacks plant a food garden borders on pretense. The "therapeutic nihilism" (Lachenal 2015, 107) that characterized the first decade of the HIV pandemic in South Africa remains a powerful affective force in the present, despite the availability of life-saving antiretrovirals (see also Le Marcis and Girard 2015). In addition, the colonial trope of the biomedical doctor doing his best under harsh conditions is often invoked in narratives of South African health care, dominated by images of burned-out junior doctors and overworked nursing staff (Pentecost and Cousins 2019).

And yet to leave the discussion there is to offer a flattened rendition of the clinic: an image of theatrical bureaucracy. Yet even bureaucracy can be empathetic (Brown 2016). Too square a focus on tools and techniques risks overlooking the relations at stake. Dr. Foster approached his nursing colleagues with empathy and a willingness to overlook small oversights in his audits.

Protocoled practice is interspersed with moments of care and relating. Staff may even engage in acts of subversive care, as in the case of Sr. Qoma dispensing formula for as long as possible so long as the tins could be ordered and no written directive contravening her practice had yet landed on her desk. Staff may go to extra lengths to care for patients, staying after hours, following up all their cases closely, or allocating deservingness of care based on estimations of a patient's background. Thus, as Julie Livingston's intricate study of a Botswana oncology ward also shows us, "moral sentiment and political efficacy are fragile in ways carefully revealed in the intimacies of care" (Livingston 2012, 91). Or, as Le Marcis and Girard (2015, 176) observed in their ethnography of South African medical services, staff may disinvest in a particular case with the justification that the patient has "defaulted" too many times. In this instance, care becomes a burden, and "withdrawing from a caring relationship is for health professionals a way to carry on working." As Akhil Gupta (2012, 24) notes, "uncaring" in such instances is integral to the functioning of the state, such that violence may be inflicted at "the very scene of care."

In sum, the pragmatics of care outlined in this chapter echo work that has shown how care has limits (Han 2012; Livingston 2012), how care has its own politics (or antipolitics) (Ticktin 2011), and how care can be viewed as a form of situated ethics (Le Marcis and Girard 2015). In Clara Han's (2012, 24) words, "care is a problem rather than a given." Drawing on the work of Veena Das (2008), Han (2012, 24) proposes that "attending to care is similar to attending to violence." Neither conforms to a script or set of practices that can be observed, audited, and evaluated. Both are deeply implicated in the moral, which Han defines "not in terms of moral judgements but in the very ways in which self is implicated with others" (24). As I came to learn, care and violence are closely imbricated in the limiting and realizing of potential in the lives of women and their children in Khayelitsha. As the subsequent chapters will show, the problem of care in conditions of injustice has important implications for women's anticipation of their future selves and the gendered selves of their children.

5 · INTERGENERATIONAL TRANSMISSIONS
The Work of Time

"Everything is possible, there's nothing impossible around," Lindiwe exclaimed during one of our conversations over the din of her large television. Lindiwe was 25 and pregnant with her second child when we met. Born in Khayelitsha, she had dropped out of high school a year before completing secondary education and gave birth to her first child shortly afterward. She started working on the factory floor of a pharmaceutical company in Cape Town and had worked there for five years on sporadic contracts. She now thought of those years as "a waste of time" and regretted not focusing on long-term goals. "Twelve hundred rand a week.[1] That was enough! On Friday I got paid and then it was the weekend. I go to the ATM and I've got money. But all that time I am playing with my life. Not anyone's life, but my life, my own thing." Lindiwe described a shift from a need for instant gratification in her younger years to the adoption of a longer-term plan that would require hard work now for rewards later. Lindiwe looked to friends whom she perceived as having done well. "They say success is a hard road: it is not achieved in a day. They are driving this Golf Five [car], they own a house in Ilitha Park,[2] a nice house, with nice things in the house, and they say 'You don't know where I am from, what path I had to walk. I had to strive. It's not that I didn't fail. I did, but I carried on. Go for education. If you want a luxury life, go for education.'" Lindiwe did not see an end to such ambition, though: "If you get to buy a house in Somerset[3] and drive a Golf, then you will want to live in Constantia.[4] You will still be hungry, hungry for other things, even if you have money. I'm not just hungry for food, I'm hungry for ideas, for improving."

Veliswa, a 30-year-old teacher, spoke similarly of a hunger for a certain kind of life for her and her children. Veliswa and her husband were both employed and sent their children to a school outside Khayelitsha. "I don't want them to experience hunger," she told me. "I want them to have options. Us at home, we didn't have options. We didn't even have a fridge. It was pap and amasi [sour milk].

That was it. I want them—if they open the fridge there is milk, cheese, eggs, bacon, everything. But I'm not just talking about hunger for food. I want them to be free, independent. Which is why I want them to get the best education ever. That is what I am working for. I want my children to have their money for themselves, to travel, to see the world."

Lindiwe was also determined that her children would not struggle as she had and described her aspirations for her children with images that denoted mobility:

> For my children, I want the best for them, the best. Not that everything they want they must have—they must know how it comes—but I'm going to take them to another level. Where there is quality, not quantity. Where everything is happening about the future. Where they can be guided. Where they can come every day with a new thing and say "Mom, I didn't know this is how it works" and I can say "Ja [Yes] my child this is how it works." I want to also know new things from them, for them to come and say "I've learnt this thing." Maybe I didn't know that, I didn't learn it at school, you see? I want them to know the technology. No one can take what is in your knowledge. Education is the best.

She recalled the words of her mother: "Ndingafundanga nje, ndizakuba fundisa abantwana bam" [I did not have the opportunity to learn, but the children will have]. Those words our great-grandmothers said to our grandmothers and our grandmothers to our mothers and my mother to me. No, I don't want to repeat that."

This chapter is about intergenerational transmissions in a different register from those at the heart of early life intervention policy. Close attention to how time is lived shakes any semblance of a patterned order of stability and disruption, particularly for reproduction and the raising of children (Johnson-Hanks 2005). To study temporality, then, one must turn to subjectivity. As Achille Mbembe (2001, 16) explains, "the time of existence and experience" consists of "an interlocking of presents, pasts, and futures that retain their depths of other presents, pasts and futures, each age bearing, altering and maintaining the previous ones." In this chapter, I describe a range of subjectivities in how people conceived of the future to illustrate the tensions between aspiration and endurance in world-making projects.

As I spent time with women and their kin during their pregnancies, our conversations inevitably turned to parents' aspirations for their children and questions of the future. Unsurprisingly, they were concerned with a very different set of future potentials than those that are the focus of first 1,000 days interventions. The women I spoke with used a range of economic, social, and spiritual strategies in the hope of realizing the futures they dreamed of, in which they had permanent jobs, a house, a car, and a good education for their children. However, not everyone believed that such goals were attainable. The disparate views of the future I encountered among my interlocutors might be described as a distribution of aspiration (see Hage 2003; Appadurai 2004). It would be easy to cast this distribution of aspiration as a question of class. Drawing on political and economic analyses of class structure in post-apartheid South Africa, one might describe some of my interlocutors as low income, a status characterized by makeshift housing, infrequent and precarious employment, and low levels of secondary school completion. Others might be categorized as emerging middle class, characterized by participation in the rental sector or property ownership, stable employment, high levels of secondary school completion, and some tertiary education (Seekings and Nattrass 2002, 2005). My participants did not fall neatly into one or other category.

THE DISTRIBUTION OF ASPIRATION

Bathandwa and her husband were ambitious. At each visit with Bathandwa, I complimented her on a new addition to her living room: new curtains, a new lounge suite, a mirror for the wall, a new cabinet for the large plasma television, a tiger-print rug. Bathandwa changed her hairstyle frequently and had her nails manicured. In response to my compliments, she would retort that her friends had just bought a house with four bedrooms, a swimming pool, and built-in cupboards in a nicer suburb. One couple she knew already owned two houses in Ilitha Park. "They've got these properties, and a Polo [car], and every time they want to take a vacation, they take a vacation. They are living the life," she sighed. Bathandwa's husband worked in the film industry, while she described herself as a housewife. They both thought that he should be moving on to something more lucrative. He had wanted to study accounting but had studied broadcasting at a technical college instead, which he regretted. "Private equity, venture capital—that's where I want to play," he mused. Like his friends, he had a property portfolio in Khayelitsha that he was working to expand. "Cape Town is expensive. Soweto or Khayelitsha, Clifton or Umhlanga Rocks[5]—across the board, Cape Town is more expensive," he shrugged. "But there is a reason why it is expensive. Because you are going to make your money. And if you don't get in now, you won't get in. It is the only province where there is still low unemployment." He lamented that he had not bought a house in Khayelitsha when he arrived in 2001, when they had cost 7,000 rand. The same house in 2015 was worth 100,000, and in Ilitha Park, houses would sell for 500,000.[6] "It's a seller's market," he concluded. Bathandwa likened her family's journey to climbing a mountain. Like Lindiwe, she believed that reaching the top was possible because others had done it. "When I go to the mountain, I always reflect on how this lifetime is very challenging, very tiring, very hectic. Some of us are faster than others. So if you see these people who can make it, it shows you, it encourages you. You can have anything in life if you sacrifice everything else for it."

Inam was also ambitious and upwardly mobile. She had a tertiary education and permanent employment. Her sister was married to a prominent councilor in Khayelitsha. When we visited her large house, I noted that it even had a home gymnasium. "The real housewives of Khayelitsha—that's what I call them," Inam said of her sister and her friends, referencing the popular reality television series that documents the lives of affluent housewives in different cities. For Inam, the next step was to become a homeowner, and she was looking for a government-subsidized house in Kraaifontein, a suburb that she preferred to Khayelitsha. "At least in Kraaifontein *they* [informal dwellers] are not right next door. Because you can't get rid of them; eventually they are going to come for lunch." Inam was clear about her aspirations: "I want to say this is *my* house, not my mother's house, *my* house."

Lindiwe made similar assertions:

> You can make of your life anything you wish. They say you must not allow the past to dictate your future. And everything that I'm doing, I must make sure I put extra time, extra effort, because I know that I wasted time. They say life begins at forty. I'm asking myself: When my life begins what assets will I have? The assets that are under my name? Can I say: "I'm governing; this is mine?" You understand? Not clothes. I'm not talking about clothes. I'm not talking about shoes. I'm talking about the qualifications [education], I'm talking about the house, and I'm talking about the car. Not a luxury life, but something that I can say: "I have worked hard for this. Here is my house guys; I'm paying a bond [mortgage]. This is my second bond. This is my car; this is my business. This is mine." You see? So this is what I am searching for. I want my own assets, my own things. I want to hold something. I want to have my life.

Lindiwe's assertion that she wanted to "have" her life illuminates a question: What does it mean to have a life? Posing this same question in the context of the United States, Lauren Berlant (2011, 117) asks "Is it to have health? To love, to have been loved? To have felt sovereign? To achieve a state or a sense of worked-toward enjoyment?" For Lindiwe, to have sacrificed, to have had patience, to have achieved a desired future for oneself and for the next generation were essential qualities for making a meaningful life. Lindiwe's desire "to govern"—to be sovereign—to "hold something" and to be able to say "here are my assets" reveals what it means to her to "have" her life—to be recognized by her society as having accomplished her goals, to have "made a life" for herself. As Ghassan Hage (2003, 16) has argued, the "key to a 'decent' society is above all this capacity to distribute these opportunities for self-realization." These opportunities are not distributed equally.

THE RECEDING DREAM

Songezwa was 33 years old when I met her. She was born in the Eastern Cape and moved to Cape Town in her late teens. She became pregnant in her final school year and failed her exams. She had since worked intermittently as a cleaner. Her first-born child went to stay with his grandmother in the Eastern Cape. Songezwa met her husband Sithembele at a meeting about funeral policies and they married when she was 26. Her second child, a girl, was born a year later. The new family built a four-room zinc shelter in Nkanini, the newest informal settlement on the edge of Khayelitsha at that time, and they have lived there since.

Songezwa would have liked to "have a house rather than a shelter," but she had little hope of moving soon. Each month was a struggle to make ends meet. It sometimes meant that the family went hungry, which made it especially difficult for Songezwa and her husband to take their antiretroviral medication. Both had been diagnosed with HIV during Songezwa's second pregnancy. Sithembele was a construction worker, but he did not have permanent employment and he was frequently at home. Often he was "waiting on an email"; a friend conducted job searches on the Internet for him. On most afternoons, we would find him watching parliamentary debates and the discussion would quickly turn to politics. "What did you do for your sixty-seven minutes?" he asked us after Mandela Day, in reference to the annual event that calls on South Africans to spend sixty-seven minutes on charitable work in memory of Nelson Mandela's sixty-seven years of activism and service. We discussed the local hospital's blanket drive I had contributed to and then I asked him about his sixty-seven minutes. He responded angrily:

> The sixty-seven minutes mean nothing to me. I worried for *myself*. For a job for *me*. I never get anything better. I can't go and busy myself with that and come back hungry. So I stayed here and cleaned my own house. I saw people painting schools on television and I thought, come to me! Do something for me! I don't blame anyone. It is the government. They are lying, lying to poor people. There is no work. Everyone is crying. The youth here are very cross. Me, I'm old already. I'm 45 and I don't have anything. I just have to wait for that time when they are going to make it right. When my daughter is finished with school she is not going to go to university because her father was not working. In the olden days, education was easy. After Standard Six, you could find work as a teacher or a nurse. Now you have to do Grade Twelve and you still won't find work.[7] During apartheid, there was order. There is no order after democracy. We sit here for many hours and there's nothing. No food. The fridge—empty. The vase—empty. Only dust.

He made a sweeping motion with his index finger and held it up to the light, as if to show us the dirt on his invisible counter.

In contrast to the hoped-for future that Lindiwe aspired to, Sithembele expressed his despairing realization that things were unlikely to get better. Having a life in this case more closely resembled "the process to which one gets resigned, after dreaming of the good life, or not even dreaming" (Berlant 2011, 177). Sithembele linked the advent of democracy to a deterioration in "order" that had allowed for the arrival of foreigners who would work for less money than South Africans. "Zimbabweans, Somalians, Nigerians, it's too much, man! Those people from Somalia—it is easy for them to open a business. The government doesn't support one of *us* opening a business," he said, gesturing to include me, Nomsa, and his wife in this statement, united by our South African citizenship. "The Nigerians do business here selling drugs. They own shoe shops in the townships, but there are drugs behind the shoes."

Sithembele expressed a surprising nostalgia for elements of the apartheid state, a phenomenon noted elsewhere in South Africa. As reported to Amber Reed (2016, 99) in the Eastern Cape, "at least life was 'certain' then: a person knew where he or she stood in the social structure and could envision the future." Jacob Dlamini (2009, 16) offers a more nuanced stance on how we might understand nostalgia for apartheid, as a way that "present anxieties [are] refracted through the prism of the past." For Dlamini, this nostalgia is less of a reactionary sentiment and more a remembrance of the social structures of solidarity that supported the struggle to end apartheid and gave rise to a vision of an equal and just future. For Sithembele, that hoped-for future had not arrived. He was at an age where the opportunity for betterment seemed already to have passed him by and the chances of his family escaping poverty seemed increasingly slim. His capacity to aspire compared to that of Lindiwe or Veliswa was severely limited, and he resigned himself to a state of "waiting until the time that they will make it right"—what Ghassan Hage (2009, 100) would refer to as the "heroism of the stuck"—a heroism that is not about what one actively achieves, but about the ability to endure, to wait out one's stuckedness.

That aspiration was unevenly distributed was more often articulated as a function of one's work or one's effort to succeed. In our conversations in the clinic waiting room, Zekiswa oscillated between sympathy for the hopelessness of others and statements that people should take responsibility for themselves. Zekiswa's position articulated the contradictions at the heart of the politics of potential at work—the ambivalent center between the call to act as a responsible, entrepreneurial agent of the self and the material circumstances that militated against that project. She would reiterate that while people's circumstances were hard, they "wasted" their chances. People were not motivated. People just sat at home. "Thirty five percent of people here think about the future," she said. "For the rest, the problem is that there is no future. That is the problem with this freedom thing. We are too free, so we are also dom [dumb]! We don't think about our future." She related her own experience: "I was also like them. How can you be motivated [to study] when you know that there are people with Matric elsewhere who are still unemployed? I spent two years not doing anything. You have to decide for yourself to change." Zekiswa explained that one needed to use the opportunities available. Her mother's employer had supported her desire to complete a course in administration. "Some of us have many chances. But many of those with chances are after drugs and alcohol. The youth want to try everything before they will change. If you ask my seven-year-old cousin, she will say that she likes this place because the elders just drink and have a good time."

Zekiswa felt that it was important for people in her community to have role models. Young people needed family support because aspiration is founded on and nourished by stability. "We need people who were once there. We can be encouraged by people who have changed in the same area. But it is the support you get at home. We don't get the love that we need. You will never hear a mother saying 'I love you' to her children. It is very rare. So we are looking for what we don't know, we are trying to catch fishes with our hands."

The capacity to realize potential is unequally distributed and shaped by historical and persistent injustices. Focused on a distant future, the politics of potential does not account for the problem of responsibility for historical injury, nor does it acknowledge the unequal circumstances that dictate intergenerational transmissions of social capital. The differential capacity to aspire between those who were more well off and those living in severely constrained circumstances manifests in differences in families' abilities to complete the necessary rituals associated with life events, such as the ability to complete marriage rituals or to properly conduct funeral rites. The naming of children, however, was one moment when parents, however rich or poor, could express aspirations for their offspring.

NAMING THE FUTURE

The Xhosa practice of naming a child in accordance with the parents' feelings or aspirations, the conditions in which the child was born, or as a message to the ancestors was important and necessary for some parents. The birth order might be reflected in the name: "Anele: it's enough." This would be the name given to the last child, but never to the first. Most of my participants chose names that evoked beauty, brightness, the future, power, greatness, recognition, or gratitude.[8] Veliswa explained:

> You can tell how the parents were feeling according to the name at the child's birth: Vuyo means joy; Nwabisa, bring joy. And also what the parents hope the child will have, or be, or become. For example, if they wish for the child to be a nurse, then her name will be Mongikazi. Nomfundo: they are wishing for that child to be educated. When we name our children, we hope that they follow their names and most of the time they do.

For Veliswa, names were imbued with potential, which also meant that great caution was required in choosing a name. Veliswa gave her first child a name that means *to dream*. She recounted how an acquaintance of hers had heard this name without knowing that she was pregnant and then later gave it to her own child. "I dreamt the name! I came up with the name!" Veliswa lamented. "She is one of those people who doesn't really dream for her kids. She stole the name." Veliswa was concerned that people were no longer taking care with naming their children:

> Young girls carry babies these days and they just name the babies. They hear the name in the clinic and they think it is a nice name. In the olden days, the naming of the child was a very important ritual. We don't just name, we think. A child's name is a big thing to Xhosa people. These days the parents are just hearing the names in the clinics and they are stealing the names. I tell the nurse to call out the surname! Because these parents steal the names. The names don't mean anything. Parents don't have a direction for their babies; they just find the name on Facebook! Each and every parent has a dream, a wish for her child. Why don't you sit down and think about the future of your child? Why don't you sit down and plan? The name can mold a child. It can destroy a child. That is why it is really important that you think. For my children, I don't steal. I think. I dream.

Choosing the correct name was seen as an important investment in a child's future, but as Veliswa observed, naming practices for the younger generation were changing with the times (see Suzman 1994; Guma 2001). As the work of Barbara Bodenhorn and Gabriele vom Bruck (2006, 2) on the anthropology of naming has shown, there is a "profound political power located in the capacity to name." Naming embeds infants in a set of relations that they will in turn influence and thus both infants and names have agency (Bodenhorn and vom Bruck 2006). The detachability of names gives them both political agency and a commodity-like value. That names could be stolen indicates their value and their recognized power in creating potential and opportunity for one's child. The exchange (or theft) of names in some way reflects the distribution of aspiration discussed here. In abject circumstances, even aspiration in the act of naming could be lost. As Veliswa uttered darkly, "I have a friend called Isiganeko, which means 'incident.' He was born on June 16, 1976.[9] If there is a war on, we will name that child Imfazwe [war]. And I know someone who named their child Indlala [poverty]. But you should never give a child a name like that. Then he will struggle for the rest of his life." As Veena Das (2015) has observed, "the name can provide a window into the way in which everyday life is imbued with the dark hues of violence, betrayal, and the corrosion of relationships" (15; see also Theidon 2015).

But more commonly naming could be an important form of future-work. My interlocutors' chosen names and the explanations they gave me of their meanings included Zusakhe (look after us), Luqhamile (brightness), Awethu (our future, our dreams, our plans), Mikhulu (greatness), Sifisosam (my wish), Lonalilamandla (the powerful), Yamihle (excellent), Mbasa (award), Iminqweno (wishes), Abukwe (to receive attention), and Ingomso (future). For many, another important place for such future-work was the church.

ALL IN GOD'S TIME

The majority of the women who participated in this study attended a Christian church. Most belonged to African Zionist congregations, but others attended Catholic, Anglican, Presbyterian, Seventh-day Adventist, or Pentecostal-Charismatic churches in Khayelitsha. I did not attend church with them and I am not able to offer comparative thoughts here about how my participants' outlooks may have differed depending on their religious affiliation, but there were important commonalities among those of Christian faith. Their aspirations and uncertainties and the future-work they did to manage them were held within another framework of time: God's time.

Aspirations, hopes, disappointments, and uncertainties were often articulated within a faith-based framework. The Christians in my study believed that church attendance and donations would help them achieve their aspirations; giving generously to the church would reap material returns (see Maxwell 2013; James 2014; and Van Wyk 2014) and offer special protection from misfortune or witchcraft. At several congregations in Khayelitsha, one attended church on the day of the week that corresponded to one's needs. At Nobomi's charismatic Christian church for example, Tuesdays were for protection against witchcraft, Thursdays were for prayers for the unemployed or imprisoned, and Fridays were "the love service" for relationship problems or desires for marriage. Many of my participants' homes were decorated with church calendars and photographs of church leaders or events with printed slogans such as "Silondozebawo" (You must protect us God).

There was a shared notion that good, God-fearing people would be rewarded. Nomsa, who described herself as Anglican, and Ndileka, who was a member of a Zionist church, agreed that in order "to have good things, one must be a good person." The notion of self-making and responsibility that Zekiswa spoke of was repeated in a cultivation of self-confidence and entrepreneurialism in the members of some churches. Songezwa and Sithembele were members of an evangelical congregation—"the kind with a keyboard," they explained. While both professed religious values, they did not extend a Christian generosity to "foreigners" who came to South Africa looking for work. Religious fervor and xenophobia were not incompatible. Rather, these seemingly conflicting attitudes were two aspects of an aspiration for a receding dream of redemption and reward for God-fearing people who had won the long fight for citizenship in the land of their birth. Both attitudes spoke to a need for order: for things (and people) to take their rightful place.

Religion was thus one available explanatory framework for life's successes and challenges and a means of creating some certainty. Disappointments or setbacks were often framed as part of "God's plan." Bathandwa had wanted to become a doctor but explained that "sometimes you want something but God has another plan for your life." Ndileka felt that her religious faith set her apart from others: "I feel it is God who going to put me where I want to be. It's only God who knows what I want, only God who can protect me from the devil. We all have challenges we are facing, but in my heart I always feel the grace of God. I can say that I am different from others."

Others found comfort in the notion Nobomi expressed that "God makes His own plan in His own time." Nobomi agreed with her mother, who said that if God wanted a certain outcome, it must be accepted. "She believes in God in every little thing," Nobomi smiled. Lindiwe similarly reasoned that "God responds in His own time, not your time. They say it is God mos [obviously] who is controlling everything."

Although witchcraft was thought to be common, it was viewed as less powerful than the will of God. "Witchcraft is strong, but if you believe in God then nothing will happen," Ndileka told me. Nomsa agreed, citing a recent dream:

> I had a dream about coins. It might mean that I will lose money in minor things, or that maybe someone is jealous that I am working now. I must be very aware not to give a person a coin if they ask to borrow money: they will use it for another purpose. They will take the five rand or ten rand and use it so that you cannot spend your money on good things. You know these people by face, but you don't know them by heart. The one who is going to hurt you is also the one who smiles at you. If you have a bad dream, you must just pray in the morning.

Nomsa's dream resonates with the entanglements of faith, witchcraft, and financial well-being that have been documented in southern Africa (see White 2001; Pfeiffer 2002; Ashforth 2005; Niehaus 2013). Apart from attending to spiritual matters, people employed several other strategies to secure their financial futures, or, in the words of the NGO worker Cebisa, make "something out of nothing."

MAKING SOMETHING OUT OF NOTHING

"Ndikwelo phulo [I'm on it, I am making an effort]. If you want something, you can do something out of nothing. In life you must have Plan A and if Plan A fails you must have Plan B. Some things are impossible, ne? Impossible. There are mission impossibles in life. Unless wena [you], you decide 'I want this future for my child' and then you have to do something out of nothing."

Cebisa's determination to do something out of nothing is contingent on an ability to navigate bureaucratic and social landscapes. Doing something out of nothing required a person to stitch together entrepreneurial opportunities and work, cobble together state provisions, balance savings and debts, and navigate bureaucracy and networks of care to gain access to other forms of support. The means available to a person and the extent to which they could engage in the reciprocities that smoothed social relations shaped their capacity to realize potential. For women like Lindiwe, financial and social capital allowed for a better stitching together of resources. Success, however, came with pressure to support one's extended family, pressure to consume, and a perception of increased vulnerability to the witchcraft of jealous acquaintances. For the less well off, doing something out of nothing was less about achieving aspirations and more about avoiding the indignity of seeking charity from neighbors. While parents articulated ambitions and hopes for their future and for the future of their children, they were all too aware of the challenges to these aspirations and of the pragmatic spirit required to overcome them.

My participants' incomes consisted of salaries (for the employed), government child support grants, Unemployment Insurance Fund benefits, money made from small entrepreneurial projects or from moneylending, and support from partners. Lindiwe's household exemplified this arrangement. Lindiwe lived in a house owned by her mother, for which her mother had a title deed.[10] The household included Lindiwe, her mother, her teenage cousin, her five-year-old son, and her recently born second child. Lindiwe managed the household's finances. "I can write down my responsibilities, each and every thing," she said. The household's income consisted of her mother's disability grant for her mild intellectual impairment (1,500 rand per month), her cousin's disability grant for her physical disability (1,500 rand per month), child support grants for each of Lindiwe's two children (700 rand in total per month), Unemployment Insurance Fund maternity benefits (1,700 rand per month for four months), her boyfriend's contributions for the baby (500 rand a month), and Lindiwe's earnings from her informal loan scheme and small businesses (variable). In addition, during holiday seasons Lindiwe rented out portable gas stoves for 100 rand per day and sold bulk bags of chicken that she bought from a local butcher. This combination of incomes was common among my participants (see also Collins et al. 2009; Du Toit and Neves 2014). With the pooled money, Lindiwe bought a monthly hamper of maize, rice, and sugar for 300 rand. She spent 200 rand per month on electricity and about 400 rand on fresh food. Other expenses included water, transport money, school fees and stationery, and cable television.

An additional expense was what Veliswa referred to as "paying the tax." The "Black tax," a term commonly used to denote the claims made by one's extended family, captures the problem of where responsibility for historical injury lands in South Africa. In this case, it is intergenerational familial ties that bear that responsibility. Scrupulous saving and self-discipline to reach "the next level" can be eroded by the obligation to help kin who are less well off. "I want my children to be whatever they want to be," Veliswa said. "Because what we are doing now—we are still working for our families, like paying a tax." Even though she and her husband were earning good incomes, they had an extended family to support. Inam also reported such obligations. Her siblings would chide her with statements such as "we'll go hungry while you still have money." She said that their demands were the reason she had not yet bought a car. Bathandwa told me that both her family and her husband's family expected support now that Bathandwa's husband had work in film. "There are expectations," she complained. "They don't see that it is still not a lot of money. His industry depends on the season. Maybe four months he is not working, then he works for two months, then we must pay the bills from four months back. Then maybe we are left with empty hands. But they don't understand that you can't look after them, that now you are married, and things have changed. Everyone expects that we must give back to them."

Apart from monthly household expenditures and "paying the tax," those with the means would engage in some form of saving, most commonly a "stokvel," or community savings club. "Everyone has a stokvel," Ndileka explained. "It starts in January and ends in the first week of December." Ndileka took part in a stokvel with her mother and three other women. Each member contributed 500 rand per month and each month one member would receive the pot of money. Ndileka used her turn to buy a dining room set for her family home in the Eastern Cape. "I believe that when I have money, I must do something that is important," she said, "so that I can say that the money I had that year, I did that and that with it." Lindiwe was also part of an annual food savings group in which each member made a monthly contribution until December, when the group bought food hampers or sheep for the holiday season.

Deborah James (2014) links the proliferation of stokvels to the growth of the middle class in South Africa and argues that they play an important role in preserving communal values. She writes that "in the midst of rapid upward swings in wealth and swift descents into impoverishment, clubs provide members with the means to communally identify and engage in reciprocal mutuality, and—guarding against the possible collapse of trust and interchange—to differentiate themselves from those of unequal means who are unable to reciprocate" (125). For my interlocutors, engaging in such reciprocities was not only a means of saving for larger expenses but was also a marker of stability and the ability to manage a household. It was a form of future-work that maintained one's dignity and inclusion in a social net of aspiration.

CREDITS AND DEBTS

In contrast with the pride that accompanied belonging to several stokvels (Nomsa participated in three), seeking loans was viewed as a sign of desperation, poor planning, and irresponsibility. As Aviwe told me, it was necessary to plan carefully to avoid seeking a loan or calling on a neighbor. That is because oomashonisa (neighborhood moneylenders; also referred to colloquially as mashonisas) charge an exorbitant interest rate of 20–30 percent.

While they never referred to themselves as oomashonisa, Lindiwe and Nobomi both lent money to people and charged a high interest rate. Nobomi was part of a group of women who worked together. Everyone contributed money at the beginning of the year. The group was divided into two teams that took turns each month to lend the money and earn interest. The clients were required to pay at the end of the month and then the increased pot of money could be loaned out again. At the end of the year the earnings were divided and the process commenced again. Nobomi earned about 20,000 rand a year with this business.[11] In the months when she was lending, our time with her would be punctuated by the sporadic arrival and exit of clients, especially on Fridays and at the end of the month, when people received wages or grants. Nobomi hid her Croxley A5 notebook with records of loans and payments under the couch. As soon as a client had left, she would motion to me to retrieve it for her so she could make a quick note. Sometimes, though, a client would miss a payment. In one case, Nobomi had not received the money after four months. "I don't like to run after people," she said. In such situations, she found it better to ask for the original loan to be returned, given that the client was unlikely to be able to repay with interest. Retrieving the money was important because it needed to be returned to the communal pot. If Nobomi could not extract it from the client, she would have to pay it herself. Her strategies in such situations included going to the client's place of employment, requesting that the client's family pay her or give her a fridge or television in lieu of payment, or asking local taxi bosses for assistance. Nobomi turned to taxi bosses only after everything else had failed because they would use unpleasant intimidating tactics that Nobomi was reluctant to elaborate on in our discussions.[12] "You have to be very firm," she shrugged. "The best thing to do when you make the loan is to take the ID [identity] book and the payment card. Then at the end of the month, you go together. He draws for you and then for himself. You don't have to shout; you don't have to do anything."

Lindiwe's experience as a moneylender had shown her how those who appeared to be most well off might sometimes be the most indebted. With the exception of cable television, Lindiwe avoided buying luxury items. "I would rather save and be patient," she said. "People end up drinking because they are going after something they can't have. If you want something, you will get it, but you must work hard and make much effort. I can see people get under pressure and they buy unnecessary things." This was especially the case in December— "the month of wasting money," as Ndileka put it. She spoke darkly about loan sharks who took advantage of those who were desperate after the excesses of Christmas. Some made advance plans for January expenses in addition to their stokvel savings. Aviwe filled her pantry with maize, sugar, flour, and nonperishable items before the start of the holiday season. She would bolt the pantry door before departing for the Eastern Cape, safe in the knowledge that there would be food for the family in January. With such forward planning, it was not necessary to seek help from moneylenders or neighbors.

Calling on neighbors for charitable assistance was a method of last resort. The women I spoke with were clear that one did not ask neighbors for help in the township. This was different from practices in the rural villages they came from. "We come from different families here," Aviwe said. "Some don't even know how to share. If you go and ask for something, especially if your husband is not working, that person will say, 'Yhu [Wow], she was here, she is struggling. Shame!'" The exclamation "shame" is commonly used in South Africa to connote pity. Aviwe's reluctance to share her problems with her neighbors was bound up with the preservation of her dignity and personhood in the eyes of her community, an observation that accords with Fiona Ross's (2010) careful research in another of Cape Town's informal settlements. Aviwe explained further: "If you go to someone and try to explain that your husband is not working, that there is no food in the house, that your baby [child] doesn't have money for [school] fees—if you take out your pain, you will hear it from someone else that you did not want to tell." Nomsa agreed: the neighbors would gossip. Aviwe had one close friend in the township she could trust. "There are few people like her. People with a heart, they are so difficult to find." If Nomsa needed help, she called on her sister. Bathandwa was frank: "I don't want to know them [the neighbors]. I just greet them in the street."

The careful cultivation of dignified relations between neighbors could, however, be quickly exposed and undone in the words and actions of a child. At Nobomi's house, her daughter Philisa's five-year-old playmate Lungi frequently joined us. Lungi was a quiet child who would hover bashfully next to her two-year-old friend. She was severely stunted for her age. "She is the same weight and height as Philisa!" Nobomi exclaimed. "When her mother told me that she will go to school soon I didn't believe her. They don't feed the baby. They like to drink." She was angry with Lungi's parents, whom she suspected of using their grant money for alcohol rather than food for the family. Lungi's father had asked Nobomi for a loan of 400 rand and although she had given it interest free, he had never returned the money. "He is working, but he doesn't buy food. It is not that they don't have the money. They just don't care.

I can't just watch him buy beers every week. It is a favor what I did. I have never seen a person who is so irresponsible like that. Can you believe that Lungi didn't have a new dress for Christmas? And she's got a [child support] grant! They are just making credits [taking loans] for alcohol. Every day they are drunk." Nobomi thought that there had to be limits to generosity in this case, but she felt compelled to help Lungi:

> The whole week, I'm maintaining Lungi. She knows when I'm going to give Philisa porridge—early in the morning she'll be here. And then Philisa says to me: 'Mommy give for Lungi too.' But sometimes I say no. If I count, this [porridge] is going to last two weeks, so I rather don't give. It is too much. On Friday they [Lungi's parents] get paid and they buy Lungi chips, but they don't share with Philisa. They are wasting my food on Lungi and then when it is their turn they don't share. On Fridays, you won't see Lungi here—she knows what is happening. So sometimes I say no, I'm not going to give her today. And then you see that she is hungry and then you feel that pain. It is not her fault. Sometimes she'll come here and sit here and just look down. I'll ask her if she is hungry, and she will nod. And then you are going to give.

As Pamela Reynolds (2000, 157) has shown in Cape Town, children will also try to make something out of nothing: they will "maximize their resources and opportunities under the circumstances in which they find themselves." Nobomi's kindness was, however, a meager resource. "I don't know how she is going to go to school. When Philisa's shoes are too small, I give them to Lungi. They won't even have a uniform for her. If she was healthy, she would have been clever, because you can see that she is clever." The social workers were aware of Lungi's circumstances and Nobomi was waiting for them to take her away.

Making something out of nothing is about the constant negotiation of financial and social opportunities and obligations and is closely tied to notions of personhood, dignity, and belonging. As Du Toit and colleagues (2007, 534) have illustrated, women in Khayelitsha are at the center of a network of "highly gendered and spatially stretched care chains" between urban and rural locations, and people are sensitive to gossip that could quickly whittle away social capital. Lungi's parents were seen as without dignity in their community: their child went hungry and did not have a new Christmas dress, they had succumbed to alcoholism, and they did little to conceal their poverty. By contrast, Aviwe carefully prepared for lean months and had chosen a trusted confidant for moments of need. Restricting one's network to those who could be trusted to maintain confidentiality did not impinge on one's dignity and it maintained an important pretext. As Fiona Ross (2015, S105) shows in the case of another of Cape Town's townships, "personhood is central to the management of debt and dependence."

NAVIGATING BUREAUCRATIC TIME

Bathandwa's lament that her husband had not yet bought another property and Songezwa's desire for a home and not just a shelter relate to state bureaucracy, a common set of obstacles that people faced as they crafted their desired futures. Achieving one's potential, making something out of nothing, or simply getting by required a fluent ability to navigate the state structures that provide access to identity documents, child support grants, title deeds, health care, and public schooling. These obstacles were more readily overcome by those with stronger social networks. Even then, bureaucracy could obstruct one's plans for months or years.

The "prize" of receiving the ID card permitted Nandipha to apply for a child support grant, open a bank account, get a learner's driving license, and apply for college. "My younger brother and my cousins got IDs before me," she said. "They were going further with their studies and I was stuck here. I didn't vote. My grandmother used to say that it doesn't matter who you vote for, as long as you voted. That paper makes a difference when you go to look for a job. My younger cousins and my brother voted but I couldn't because I didn't have an ID. It was painful. I felt like I was nothing."

However, in South Africa, an ID is not enough to register for state grants, elective public health care, subsidized housing, and public education. One also needs pay slips and a proof of address. People navigated these requirements in different ways. It was common for women who were applying for a child support grant to travel from Khayelitsha to the Eastern Cape, where officials were less likely to enforce rules about declaring income. It was generally agreed that it was best not to disclose any informal work when making the application. At the same time, those seen to be abusing the system were frowned upon. The money was meant for those who were "suffering," as Ndileka put it, and not for those "whose husbands are working." In Khayelitsha, child support grants were frequently reallocated to more pressing concerns (see also Du Toit and Neves 2009). For example, Bathandwa's child support grants supported her mother, who did not yet have a pension. Child support grants were often drawn directly by another family member (usually a grandparent) to spend on children who were living with them in the Eastern Cape.

For public health care and public schooling, South African citizens are eligible to access facilities nearest to their place of residence. Those who wished to access schools and hospitals in other areas would try to obtain a document that could demonstrate proof of address in qualifying suburbs, such as a police affidavit that they resided with family in the area, despite this not being the case. Many women preferred to deliver their babies at the secondary-level maternity hospital in Mowbray, an affluent suburb closer to Cape Town's central business district. "You need an address," Veliswa explained to me. "That is what is tricky about our democracy. It's been twenty years but now still this!" Veliswa viewed the differential access based on where one lives as discriminatory because residence in Cape Town is still highly segregated along racial lines. "I think you should be able to go where you like, where you feel safe. I had a friend living in Mowbray, and I had to say that she was my cousin and that I was living with her. I had to make an affidavit. And then no problem, everything was perfect." Lindiwe was anxious to find an address in Cape Town's southern suburbs so that she could enroll her son in primary school there. She obtained proof of address for Kenilworth, another affluent suburb, through one of her teachers, who volunteered to attest that Lindiwe was resident at her household. "You must take your children to White schools," Nomsa said. "All of the children in my family were taken to White schools. That's why everyone speaks English. I don't want to be blamed when my child is older: if he is eighteen and he can't speak English, who is he going to blame?" As Mark Hunter (2015) has observed, schooling choice in contemporary South Africa is closely tied to racially inflected perceptions of social and symbolic capital. There was a common desire for children to attend school in Cape Town's affluent areas where English was the language of instruction. Inam, who had attended a formerly Whites-only public school in Cape Town, wanted to send her children to private schools "for an education that not just anyone could afford."

Property acquisition was also an exercise in patience. Bathandwa and her husband had bought a house in 2007 from a woman on the government housing list. They obtained an affidavit from the police as proof of payment and had since been trying to obtain a title deed. Bathandwa moved into the property for a few weeks while it was being renovated in the hope that the officials might come by with the deed in that time as promised. "They say that if you are not at the house, they are going to give a title deed to whoever is there at the time," she said. She had heard stories of people coming back to their tenants to find that the tenant had been given the title deed. "You can go away and come back, and this person says, 'I have a title deed, this is my house now.'" The perception that housing officials were corrupt and might hand out title deeds to someone other than the rightful owners was common and perhaps not entirely unfounded (Rubin 2011). For Bathandwa and her husband, they had been "waiting for the state" (Oldfield and Greyling 2015) to provide a title deed for longer than the national average time of around five years for those who had been allocated houses by the government. Negotiating housing allocation and property acquisition thus depended on a person's ability to navigate a state bureaucracy that was both inefficient and potentially corrupt. As Colin Hoag (2013, 411) has described in his ethnography of the South African Department of Home Affairs, "powerful bureaucracies control and contort time." As my participants' battles with identity documents, health care, schooling, and housing made clear, bureaucracy could stretch out time and delay the future.

INTERGENERATIONAL TIES

In the context of reinvigorated scientific understandings of the intergenerational transmission of health and disease, few researchers have attended to how people conceptualize the intergenerational and strive toward betterment for subsequent generations. In this chapter I have illustrated some of those means of intergenerational investment. Far from the epigenetic imaginaries of intergenerational health, ideas about and aspirations for the future were embodied in infants' names and configured by bureaucratic and religious time, by a nostalgia for a past order, or by the seasonal ebbs and flows of debt and credit. Intergenerational investments were sought amid variable constraints as well as gendered and generational tensions. As research on the consequences of social protection on intergenerational ties in South Africa has shown, grant provisions to specific categories of persons (women and the elderly) reconfigure networks of care and dependency in ways the state does not acknowledge (Moore and Seekings 2019). Women are the heads of households. they are the key recipients of social grants, and they are the primary caregivers for the young, the old, and the infirm (Hatch and Posel 2018; Mkhwanazi and Manderson 2020). Intergenerational claims obligate one to support one's kin, and these claims are gendered.

The gendered securing of the future conjured by first 1,000 days policies amplifies already existing social configurations in which future-making is gendered work. But the distant focus on potential at the heart of those policies does not accord with the potentialities that shaped affect and ambivalence for my interlocutors, most notably the potential for violence.

6 · AMBIVALENT KIN
On Gender and Violence

Nobomi answered the door in ripped jeans and a T-shirt that said "Every generation has its struggle." On the back, it said "My struggle should not be my children's struggle." She was heavily pregnant and expecting to deliver her baby soon. She had bad news. The previous Monday, around noon, Nobomi had been in her room with two-year-old Philisa. Nobomi's sister was in the bathroom. They heard four shots being fired into their kitchen. When they went to the kitchen to see what had happened, they found a man dead on the kitchen floor, next to the refrigerator. They did not know him. A neighbor had called the police, who arrived shortly afterward and took statements. "The police were here asking us questions," Nobomi said, "but we didn't see nothing. They made as though we know." She described how they had been told not to touch or move the body; the police said that everything would have to be left as is until the forensics unit had arrived. The forensics team had not come until around 5 P.M., some five hours later. "Forensics took pictures, they took statements and they put some stickers under the gunshots," Nobomi recalled. The body was finally removed at 7 P.M. Nobomi said that she had asked the police how a body could lie in someone's house all day when it was not even the house of the victim's family, but they had responded that their hands were tied. "That day, I thought I was going to deliver," she said. Another neighbor had helped them clean up afterward. "We know the family of the guy, but no one came to check the mess," Nobomi said. "In the fridge we have bullet holes; in the cupboard as well." She pointed them out: two bullet holes in the kitchen cupboards, one in the side of the refrigerator, and one that was visible when Nobomi opened the refrigerator and pointed to the hole at the back. The fridge was empty. The bullet holes were marked with small measurement stickers so the viewer could intuit the size of the hole from the photographic image. Nomsa, in her pragmatic fashion, asked if the fridge was still working. "Yes," Nobomi answered, "but I don't think that it will work for a long time. My grandfather says that we must change this fridge and the cupboard doors, because every time we look at these, we are going to have memories." When I asked how Philisa had responded to this, Nobomi replied, "She said, 'Mama, these people are going to come back, and they are going to shoot us.' The counselor said that before she falls asleep, we must whisper in her ear that nothing will happen." Nomsa explained this practice: "It's like when someone in the family dies, we normally let the child know. Siyamhlebele endlebeni—to speak in a baby's ear, so that they forget for now. One whispers 'Akukho nto izakwenzeka' [Nothing will happen]."

This is one account of a single day in the first 1,000 days of two-year-old Philisa's life. It is a fragment, in the words of Veena Das (2007, 5): "unlike a sketch that may be executed on a different scale from the final picture one draws, or that may lack all the details of the picture but still contain the imagination of the whole, the fragment marks the impossibility of such an imagination." It is a difficult but necessary task to portray how violence could undermine my interlocutors' aspirations. For them, living in anticipation of a hopeful future coexisted with the fearful anticipation that that potential future would be cut short. While my interlocutors' aspirations and hopes are about the future in a representational sense, these accounts illustrate the future in its affective sense: the ordinary anticipation that structures everyday life. They are recorded here not for their spectacular nature, but because their comprehension is central to an understanding of how the women I worked with in Khayelitsha viewed and related to the future in ways that illuminate a temporal limit to the politics of potential as conceived in early life intervention programs. Perceptions of both potential and risk were also deeply gendered in ways that are not apprehended in policy.

GENDERED FUTURES: "DON'T GIVE ME A BOY"

Nobomi recounted the story as a terrible event, but of a kind that happened frequently in Khayelitsha. She placed the man's death in the context of gang activities in her area and recalled some of the gang fights over the weekends before the murder. The deceased man, Nobomi understood, had been threatening rival gang members in the week before his death. His brother had also been attacked and had sustained severe head injuries. Nobomi told me that when the man's mother had found out about his death, all she had said was, "This time, my baby didn't do nothing."

Nobomi feared that her brother Dlame would suffer the same fate. Dlame, who often came and went during our visits with Nobomi, arrived home just as she finished recounting this event. Nobomi motioned to him to lift his Ray-Ban sunglasses to show us his most recent injury. He lifted the glasses to reveal a fresh scar across his right eye, about ten centimeters long, sutures still in situ. Nobomi and her mother had pleaded with him not to take revenge on a rival gang for this attack.

Over the course of fifteen months, I spent significant time at Nobomi's home and met everyone in her household. However, my interactions with Dlame had been limited to greetings as he came and went from the house. In keeping with the matrifocality that has historically characterized and still characterizes many households in the Western Cape as a result of apartheid's migrant labor systems, Nobomi lived in a household of mostly women. And as with most women-headed households, it was women's resources that supported its members. Like many households in Khayelitsha, the members of Nobomi's household traveled between a rural homestead and the township at least a few times a year. Nobomi's mother was a formally employed breadwinner. Her father was deceased. Nobomi, her older brother, and her sisters engaged in various forms of informal work and did all of the domestic work in the house. Nineteen-year-old Dlame was mostly left to himself.

"He is one of the skollies," Nobomi said. A skollie, as Elaine Salo (2018, 182) explains it, has a "ruffian identity" as a "non person, the stranger who exists beyond the boundaries of the local community," a person who "bring[s] shame to their own mothers and households" and presents a material threat to their own families and communities. Nobomi told me that when he was 13, Dlame had joined a local gang and formed a drug habit:

Dlame is smoking tik [methamphetamines]. On weekends, he doesn't sleep at home, and there are a lot of reports coming. He doesn't want to go to school. He can go for a week, two weeks, and he doesn't take a bath. Because of that tik. He was not like that. But ever since he started smoking tik, he doesn't wash, even his teeth. We've tried everything. Now we just leave him. If he doesn't come home, we don't look for him. We used to stress, but now if he is not here, we just leave it. If he is back, he is back.

Nobomi said that he had begun to steal to fund his drug addiction. "He takes people's stuff. He steals something here that we are not going to notice now—maybe the CDs, or the CD player, or a charger—the small stuff. He takes my necklaces, my earrings. I can't leave anything lying around." Nobomi repeatedly complained that Dlame ate the lion's share of the household's groceries:

Sometimes the babies don't have anything to eat because he is wasting my babies' food. He eats alone because he knows that he is going to eat more. Not two eggs: he wants four. I must hide food. Maybe I want to buy sausages, but they come in packs of thirteen. The babies will eat one and the rest will go in the fridge. When I look again, they are gone. I ask why he doesn't just leave one for the child. He says he doesn't have a child, so he doesn't think about it. These fights with my brother are stressing my mom. But I have kids now. I must buy more now, and he is going to keep wasting and then there are two babies crying for me. He doesn't understand, and if he does, he doesn't care.

Nomsa too had a skollie in the family. Siseko was her nephew. Nomsa and I would see him periodically at a busy intersection in Khayelitsha, where he would hang out on the corner with a few others. Nomsa would wring her hands and say: "There's Siseko! He's not in school again!" Siseko, her mother's first grandson, was born in 1994. Nomsa was ten years old at the time. "I remember that my mother was very excited, although I was very little. Everybody was excited because they had freedom and it was their first time to vote." It was equally exciting that Nomsa's sister had given birth. In 2010, Siseko's mother was diagnosed with tuberculosis. "I was the one who was looking after her," Nomsa explained. "She was sick for a long period of time. Her doctor was confused. She stopped the medication because she didn't know what the problem was. Instead of getting better she was getting worse. We changed the hospitals, but every time it was the same. On 6 July 2010, she died." Nomsa made all of the arrangements for the funeral, which took place in the Eastern Cape. Siseko was 13 years old and orphaned. In Cape Town, he started to do the "wrong things," Nomsa said. "He started to rob people." Nomsa's family attributed this to drug use, so they sent him to the Eastern Cape where he could stay with his grandmother and attend the local school. Siseko did not complete his schooling and came back to Cape Town to live with one of Nomsa's sisters. Every time Nomsa and I passed him on the street, she would shake her head and talk about how bad it was to drink and smoke tik— how Siseko had met the wrong crowd and joined the gangs.

I learned of Siseko's death at the age of 21 in August 2015. It was a Monday morning like many others in Khayelitsha, characterized by a slow collection of reports of the weekend's activities from participants, frequently including reports of incidents of crime. Siseko had been relaxing at a friend's house the previous morning when the gathering was interrupted by the police on a drug raid. The police allegedly demanded that everyone lie down to be searched for drugs. Nomsa contended that Siseko was terrified of arrest and attempted to run away. The witnesses at the scene reported that a White policeman had shot Siseko four times as he fled and that he had fallen in the sand between two shacks. The police had called an ambulance, and when it arrived, the paramedics had certified him dead. No drugs were found. His body was cordoned off awaiting forensics, and the family first became aware that he had died when his aunt came across the forensic scene on her way home from Sunday church. She alerted the family immediately so they could intercept the other children and take them on an alternative route home. The policeman in question was not suspended. "We thought he might come to apologize," Nomsa said, "but nothing." Nomsa's five-year-old son kept asking what had happened to Siseko. Nomsa could not answer.

Both Nomsa and Nobomi wished for girl children and, like many of the other women I spoke with, expressed fear about raising boys. Nobomi gestured to Dlame, who had dropped out of school at age 14, and her cousin Sihlobo, who had been expelled from school after he had allegedly attempted to stab a teacher. Fifteen-year-old Sihlobo, Nobomi said, was even more of a disappointment than Dlame, because he had been given so much. "They live in a better house, they drive a better car, and on weekends they eat out. He's wearing brands—Carvela, Red Jeans, nice jackets. It's such a disappointment." Like Dlame, Sihlobo was using drugs. His mother bought him expensive clothes and tablet computers, which he sold for drug money, claiming that they had been lost or stolen.

Nobomi was very glad when she delivered another girl. She gave the following explanation:

> In this environment we live in, boys get influenced by the wrong things too easily. Small boys from the age of twelve are smoking, drinking, starting to be skollies. Girls, they don't walk around; they know what time to be home. If a boy is growing up nicely, the others will laugh at him, because few boys don't drink and smoke. It's not easy growing a baby, and then he's a skollie. I mean if you don't have food you must try to get him something to eat when he is a baby and then at the end of the day, he is a skollie! If your child is a skollie, he might beat you in your own house. So you are also at risk. They can come and catch him and kill him right in front of you. The community stands up: they burn them and they beat them. You know what happens if you buy something, like maybe a DVD, from my brother? Your house will be on fire. Your house is going to be burnt down.

Nobomi was asked by her distressed aunt to take Sihlobo to the drug center at the local clinic, where he tested positive for methamphetamines and cannabis. His mother was distraught. "I've wasted enough [resources] hoping that Sihlobo is going to be someone or something one day," she told Nobomi. "I don't want to waste any more money. Rehab will be expensive." Sihlobo had been raised by his grandmother in the Eastern Cape, then sent to his mother for high school. Now faced with the threat of being sent back to the Eastern Cape, Sihlobo had cried, but his mother retorted: "What about my tears? Growing a baby is not easy."

Nomsa agreed that a boy child was a risk because he might join a gang. "We don't live in peace now," Nomsa said. "And I don't know if in ten years' time it is going to be better or worse. My son will be a teenager in ten years; maybe he will stop going to school and be a skollie. If I have another one, I want a baby girl."

Inam also lived with a household of women—her mother and her sisters and their girl children—and she echoed the desire for a girl. To her ultrasonographer's surprise, Inam was patently upset when she found out that her unborn child was a boy. "I was so distraught, I shrieked. She had to console me," she recounted. "I couldn't eat. I kept thinking: scans can lie. I just need to keep that thought in my mind. I kept saying that if it is a boy, I'm going to turn him into a girl. I'm going to buy him pink shirts and everything. I thought it was a girl, I still think it is a girl in my head. When I give birth and they tell me it's a boy, then I'll believe." Inam would coo at her niece and tell her to "play with Aunty's tummy, so maybe it will be a girl." The only boy living in her household was her cousin who had come to live with them. "Everyone else is living with their mom, it must be hard for him," she said. "His mother was never very affectionate."

Inam's observations—that boy children might be cast out by their own mothers—shaped her feelings of ambivalence during pregnancy about raising a boy. When she gave birth to a baby boy, she told me that she had accepted the situation, but her anxiety was still palpable:

> I'll just sit and pray that he doesn't start smoking and getting into gangs. A girl, she might bring a baby, but a boy—he can kill someone, or steal your stuff. This person is in your house. And then you think: you gave birth to this man—he couldn't kill a man in cold blood. . . . You wish you could pick up and go somewhere until they are old enough. There's no way that a child will be perfect, but you just have to pray that he'll keep making the right choices. At the end of the day, if he doesn't, then it is his choice.

Like Inam's thoughts of picking up and go somewhere else, women discussed the possible mitigation strategies they might deploy to protect a boy child: for example, sending the child to live with grandparents in the rural homestead, or ensuring that he was enrolled at a school outside the township if the child were to stay in Khayelitsha. The fears women expressed about raising boys during pregnancy did not mean that they would not love their sons. Rather, their honest reflections reveal intimate truths that point to the specific contours of maternal ambivalence in a context of matrifocal families and migrant labor systems, decreasing marriage rates, the HIV epidemic, and high levels of gender discord and gender-based violence.

Women's discussions about having girls or boys also reflected their perceptions that daughters would be more likely to care for them later in life. These women were all either married or in relationships with men, and they spoke about their children's futures in ways that repeated traditional gender roles. While they acknowledged that male partners and grandparents might dote on a son, they believed that girls had a better chance of finishing school, supporting their families, and achieving their own (and their mothers') aspirations (see also Lee 2009). Bathandwa was forthright:

> There were four of us and my mother; no father figure. The men—they work for themselves and only contribute when it is helpful for them. Even if a girl is married, she must go back home. The men, they forget about where they came from

most of the time. But for us women, we must see that our mother is eating. The mother is everything. She is the one who supported you through all of your ups and downs. So you can't just ignore it when she says she doesn't have food, you must bring something. Boys—they don't worry, they don't care. You are blessed if you have boys who care for their mothers, but they are few. Most women though, they know that you can't just ignore, because when you were growing up you knew that your mother raised you, and now she doesn't have the strength. So you are raised to give back. Responsibility for your mother and your children, it is the same. You are in this position because of her. These ones [the children] can't do anything and at a certain stage, maybe they'll be the ones looking after you.

Just as Sihlobo's mother was tired of "wasting" her money on hoping that Sihlobo would be "something or someone one day," so did women such as Bathandwa articulate the hope that daughters would reciprocate the care they had received when their mothers needed help in later life. Intergenerational care in this context was thus less shaped by notions of future physical or mental health and more by notions of intergenerational duty, and the expectation was that it was daughters who were likely to fulfill such obligations.

The commonalities among my interlocutors' views suggests a "regime of subjectivity," in the words of Mbembe and Roitman (1993, 324), "a shared ensemble of imaginary configurations of 'everyday life,' imaginaries which have a material basis; and systems of intelligibility to which people refer in order to construct a more or less clear idea of the causes of phenomena and their effects, to determine the domain of what is possible and feasible, as well as the logics of efficacious action." As psychologist Lou-Marie Kruger (2020) has argued, research with pregnant and low-income women in South Africa has focused on behavior and neglected women's subjective experiences of pregnancy. The regimes of subjectivity that inform parenting for some of my interlocutors in Khayelitsha included an ambivalence about having boys, a departure from older patrilineal frameworks that prized male children (Radcliffe-Brown and Forde 1950). This ambivalence does not preclude care or intergenerational investment. Understanding ambivalence in this case offers productive possibilities for thinking about kinship (Peletz 2001; Rigg and Peel 2016) by offering insights into how maternal subjectivities are deeply informed by present personal circumstances, past experiences, and calculations of potential futures.

As Elaine Salo (2018, 162) documented in another Cape Town township, there is a "process of racial and gendered exclusion through the lifecycle" of men and boys at work here, alongside chronic exposure to systemic violence. This has uncomfortable resonances with long-standing racialized narratives of violence in South Africa (Graham 2012), but as Steffen Jensen (2008) observed in his study of criminality in Cape Town, the extent to which such stereotypes influence people's conception of themselves and their kin is not insignificant.

Gender studies in South Africa have devoted significant attention to the link between violence and masculinity in an effort to understand the country's high rates of gender-based violence and the impact of that violence on the HIV epidemic (Morrell et al. 2013). While research initially focused on understanding men's gendered practices, more recently there has been recognition of the need to research women's subjectivities to understand women's ambivalence about and negotiation of relations with men, and how a gender order characterized by patriarchy and a tacit acceptance of violence is reproduced and maintained (Jewkes and Morrell 2012). As in Jewkes and Morrell's study (2012) in the Eastern Cape, the women I worked with navigated gender relations in one of three ways: some were subservient to men, accepting the cultural capital that came with surrendering and living in submission in accordance with custom; a few espoused a modern femininity that spurned marriage and cohabitation in favor of independence (although this frequently meant living in their mother's household); and some occupied a middle ground, tolerating a culture of men in power while seeking out relations based on respect and avoiding violence. Women's ambivalence about and negotiation of relations with men in this case reflects "affective transmission[s]" (Meinert and Grøn 2020, 581) of a gender construct of men (and boys) as predisposed to violence (see also Helman and Ratele 2016). In contrast to the anticipatory logic offered by early life interventions, for childbearing women in Khayelitsha anticipated futures were closely tied to the fraught negotiations of gender relations. Adams and colleagues (2009, 247) define anticipation as the "palpable effect of the speculative future on the present". In this view, anticipation is part of an affective state, "*a way of actively orienting oneself temporally*" (247, emphasis in original). For the women I worked with, anticipation was structured by dominant gender norms, ambivalent kinship, and fears of violence, and this was often expressed as a concern about the fate of young boys. This ambivalence in turn is implicated in the social exclusion of boys and men in a context where masculinities are partly shaped by legacies of state violence and partly by both men and women's reproduction of hegemonic masculinity and gender norms (see Morrell et al. 2013; Salo 2003; Talbot and Quayle 2010; Hunter 2010; and Mkhwanazi 2014).

The focus on women of reproductive age in DOHaD interventions mirrors other social forms of investment and exclusion, in which men and young boys often fall outside the public health gaze and outside protective networks of kin and community. This is not to suggest that interventions should adopt frames that fall into equally problematic reifications of men and masculinity, as work in gender studies (Morrell 1998; Connell 2005; Ratele 2016) and public health (Dworkin et al. 2012; Fleming et al. 2014; Gibbs et al. 2015) has cautioned against. Rather, the task is to question what is reproduced and how. The empirical material offered here highlights the need to understand the operation of gender in the framing of futures in more capacious terms: not simply as an identity, which leads to simplistic frameworks of young women who should be "good mothers," but also as a force that patterns interactions and shapes kinship relations and as social structure that ironically is re-created in the very institutions, systems, and practices that purport to work toward a better future for all. The anticipatory logic of the first 1,000 days framework overlooks complex gender dynamics. It also stands in contrast to the affective state of anticipation that characterizes everyday life in volatile spaces.

AFFECT AND THE CITY

The watchfulness, vigilance, and anxiety that structured women's lives in Khayelitsha were revealed in fragments, encounters, and anecdotes that evoked fear and apprehension. One day, it was the burned carcass of a car on a route Nomsa and I drove daily. "They hijack the car, take the parts, then set it alight so it can't be identified," Nomsa explained. "If you're in a hijacking, don't look at them," she told me pragmatically. "Just look at the number plate. If you look them in the eye, they're going to kill you. You just look at the ground and look at the number plate and put it in your head and then later write it down." Another day, Nobomi's sister tearfully reported that she had been mugged on the way home from school. Another day, a child was injured in gang crossfire at the school gates. Another day, Nomsa and I encountered a group of young men sauntering slowly down the road, obstructing our vehicle. "I know one of those guys, they won't bother us," Nomsa said. Later that day she learned that the group had robbed an elderly man in the park. She expressed bitter disappointment in this young man, whom she had known since he was a child. On yet another occasion, Bathandwa told me about a friend's death. His car had broken down on the N2 highway between Khayelitsha and the airport. While he waited for assistance, he was hijacked and stabbed in the leg by a group of men. He had been receiving treatment for cancer. "He had to stop the chemo while the wound was healing, and then he died," Bathandwa said. "He was so young, so young."

None of the women I engaged with had private transport; they all walked from their homes to the closest taxi stop or train station. For many women, this short walk was a time of extreme vulnerability. Nursing staff told of pregnant patients stabbed on their walk to the clinic. Khanyiswa had witnessed several robberies on her morning walk to the train to get to school. "It is not safe, especially in the morning. I miss Jo'burg [Johannesburg]. The safety. I miss the safety. Here you can't walk with your phone. There is crime in Jo'burg, but not like this." Inam recounted two incidents on her early morning walk to catch a taxi. "The first time, I saw him walking towards me, so I ran back and went around the other way. I got to the taxi with him still running towards me." The second time, during early pregnancy, she had become aware of a man hiding at the taxi rank as she approached. Fortunately, the taxi arrived and she jumped in. "I was almost robbed; I was almost robbed. There's no place where you feel safe," she said. Her constant anxiety worsened significantly during her pregnancy. Bathandwa had stopped attending church on Wednesday nights because she felt unsafe walking home: "All over there are young guys using tik, and they are looking for a target." She was assaulted for her phone and her wallet a few months after the baby's birth. "It is dangerous to walk around," Zekiswa said. "You leave your house, and you fear what you have left behind. If your child is coming home from school, you worry that he may be kidnapped." Lindiwe expressed the same anxiety: "They wait outside the high school; they wait for the students to come out. And you don't even know what is going on. You will just see the bricks coming. You are worried about the crossfire. Your child doesn't know anything; he is just carrying his bag, thinking he's going to phone his mom now and then the brick comes. Imagine. The brick just comes straight at him and knocks him down."

Lindiwe described her ritual for walking home in the evening: "If I walk across the bridge, I walk ten steps, then I observe. I walk another fifteen, and then I observe. Before I come into the house, I observe, then I go around the house, then I come in and I lock the door." Nights, weekends, and public holidays were perceived as especially dangerous times to be outside. "You don't want to go out on the weekends," Lindiwe said. "In the park, there is warfare. They're carrying guns. Everyone is drinking and people lose their balance. I'd rather stay here. I lock that gate and I stay here. If you want music, it is here. TV, it is here." On public holidays more alcohol would be consumed. "A lot of things happen at that time," Anele said. "They stab each other; they fight a lot." She had lost a cousin on Christmas Day in 2005. "That is why we stay inside on that day."

Life in Khayelitsha seemed tempered by a rhythm of self-imposed curfews and rituals. Life was lived in chronic anticipation. In the context of such volatility, women often shared a sentiment that one should "live for today." As Bathandwa explained,

> These kinds of things make me think on my toes. Don't think of the future, just think of now. The Bible says that we must not worry about tomorrow, because tomorrow will worry about itself. Enjoy today. Live today. You don't know what you're going to miss. If you keep the bread for tomorrow, you don't know if you will have tomorrow. Most of us, even myself, we leave things for tomorrow. But life is surprising. It's like, ah! Here's a new thing. You thought you knew life, but then life surprises you with something else. You thought you are living life, but then it leaves you, just like that. You don't have that life you thought you had.

CORROBORATIONS

As I perused the Khayelitsha Commission of Inquiry's report on crime and policing in Khayelitsha, I found testimonies that closely resembled the reports of violence and crime that featured almost daily in my conversations in Khayelitsha. The incidents I heard about were not sensational exceptions. Khayelitsha residents were the victims of frequent crimes and they were exposed to high levels of violence against others. The commission's full report and findings provided evidence that corroborated my participants' stories.

Formed in 2012 and concluded in August 2014, the Khayelitsha Commission included testimonies from activists, community leaders, and residents who attested to the high rates of violent crime, gang activity, vigilantism, and homophobic and xenophobic violence in the township. As she presented the commission's findings to a conference audience in Stellenbosch in November 2014, Justice Catherine O'Regan, who co-led the commission with Advocate Vusumzi Pikoli, described ineffective detective services, understaffed police services, and significant underreporting of crime in Khayelitsha. O'Regan reported that crime statistics from Khayelitsha were largely unreliable and that two-thirds of crimes went unreported. Even so, Khayelitsha had the highest rate of reported murder, sexual assault, grievous bodily harm, and aggravated robbery in the country. O'Regan's conclusion was unflinching: "There is no doubt that if you grew up in Khayelitsha, you have seen acts of vigilantism. The level of postviolence deep trauma in Khayelitsha is enormous."

The Khayelitsha Commission's report also presented a pertinent example of how a host of social ills are increasingly explained in terms of epigenetics and transgenerational transmission. The report included expert testimony from Prof. Pumla Gobodo-Madikizela, a psychologist with expertise on intergenerational trauma. She suggested that for Khayelitsha, "the culture of violence [has] been transmitted from the past, and continues to transform identities and to play out both as cultural memory and collectively shared traumatic memory" (quoted in Khayelitsha Commission 2014, 344). Her assessment coheres with long-standing research in South Africa on social work, literary theory, and the psychology of intergenerational trauma (Gobodo-Madikizela 2016; Adonis 2016; Hoosain 2013; Mengel and Borzaga 2012). In contrast, Dr. David Harrison offered a biological explanation for the "transgenerational transmission of violence"; he argued that it is related to the "epigenetic effects of harmful environments." He explained that early life was critical for one's life trajectory and spoke of "the developing understanding of the effect the environment has on our epigenetic constitution, that environmental factors affect our genes" (quoted in Khayelitsha Commission 2014, 135).

The first 1,000 days provides one lens for viewing a turn to epigenetic frameworks to make sense of the "biology of history" (Landecker 2016, 19) in South Africa. That these ideas entered a legal report as part of expert testimony on the effects of violence on children in Khayelitsha in 2014 illustrates their explanatory currency for a host of social ills. This is just one of the popular and institutional contexts that have adopted epigenetic frameworks for heredity and the concept of the intergenerational transmission of risk in the framing of future outcomes.

SOCIAL TRANSMISSIONS

The concepts of epigenetic trauma and transgenerational transmission have also been articulated in South Africa's popular press. These ideas appeared in two publications in 2016 that took the causative chain one step farther: they linked early life malnutrition to a predisposition toward violence in adulthood. In *Gang Town*, journalist Don Pinnock (2016, 170) contended that "delinquency" on the Cape Flats may be secondary to what he calls "epigenetic development disorder" and that the intractability of gang culture is potentially linked to "early epigenetic trauma" that may be "ultimately irreversible" (173). Pinnock's book covers the historical beginnings of gang culture in Cape Town, the present-day local and transnational criminal and corporate networks that constitute it, the inequality and poverty that help perpetuate it, and the possible interventions to consider across a range of sectors—a worthy project in need of attention. It is however noteworthy that the language he deployed to explain the phenomenon of gang violence includes epigenetic frameworks and that the mother is again a key site of intervention. *Gang Town* described the first 1,000 days as a period of plasticity when a stress-free prenatal and postnatal environment (again circumscribed to the mother) can have epigenetic effects that promote self-regulation.

A similar argument in the popular press the same year *Gang Town* was published linked malnutrition and violence. The author wrote, "Research on the links between hunger and violence found that chronic malnutrition in early life may permanently damage the brain's impulse-control mechanism, resulting in adults who have a strong predisposition to react violently in social situations. . . . What this implies is that many malnourished South African children are having their brains permanently rewired to predispose them to violence" (Ledger 2016). While the authors of these publications wished to highlight the structural factors that underlie South Africa's endemic violence, their arguments included a dangerous turn toward deterministic understandings of the impacts of early life factors for future health and life outcomes.

The descriptions of everyday life Bathandwa and others shared included a high degree of what the scientific and popular literature would refer to as "prenatal stress." The effects of early life stressors on future health outcomes are a significant area of inquiry in the fields of DOHaD and epigenetics (Mulligan 2016), including whether early life interventions that target interactions between genes and environments, parental investment, neurodevelopment, and self-regulation might prevent violence in future generations. While the experiences of Bathandwa and others show how material and structural conditions create an adverse environment, the most frequent site for early life intervention is the mother herself, who is called to act as a *"buffer"* against this adversity (Morgan 2014, 105, italics in original). A significant body of work, much of it conducted in Khayelitsha, thus focuses on interventions aimed at improving maternal attachment and care (Cooper et al. 2009; Tomlinson 2012) as a strategy for preventing future violence (Ward et al. 2014; Skeen et al. 2015). Scientists are even interested in the possibility that genetic and epigenetic biomarkers could be used in the future to prescribe psychosocial interventions (Morgan et al. 2017).

Interventions that target maternal behavior are perceived as the most feasible means of improving outcomes in the context of the seeming impossibility of ameliorating the socioeconomic inequalities that shape early life adversity. Kasia Tolwinski (2019, 157), who studied neuroscientists' understandings of poverty and adversity, refers to this as a "scientific sociological imagination" that acknowledges structural factors but still focus interventions at the individual or molecular level. Dorothy Roberts's (2016, 124) diagnosis in this case is terse: "The scientists' aim is no longer to understand how unequal power arrangements inflict biological injuries. Their aim becomes to evaluate individuals' biological fitness to withstand exposure to unequal social environments."

In light of notions of the transgenerational inheritance of trauma, the question of the effects of violence on relationships becomes an altogether different political question. The fact that the Khayelitsha Commission's report on crime and police inefficiency draws on expert testimonies about the epigenetic effects of harmful environments and the transgenerational transmission of trauma and violence requires attention. It is an important example of how emergent scientific concepts such as DOHaD, epigenetics, and the first 1,000 days come to be a part of popular understandings of social outcomes. There is cause for caution against the unreflexive uptake of epigenetics as an explanatory model in the policy and public spheres. The commission's report attempts to highlight the important difference between the future outcomes for those who grow up in safe suburbs and those who grow up exposed to high levels of crime. Similarly, scientists and journalists are well-meaning in their searches for routes to intervention for endemic violence in South Africa. However, to speak of the transgenerational transmission of violence, the permanent rewiring of brains, or epigenetic trauma risks slipping into determinism. The causative leap that might be made between early life experiences and adult violence abstracts individuals from their social circumstances and by virtue of the slippage between "early life" and "intrauterine life" (Mansfield 2017) invites scrutiny of the mother.

In sum, the politics of potential engenders a turn toward deterministic, essentialist, or biologized notions of inheritance that concentrate intervention efforts on the maternal body. A focus on the broader infrastructures that shape the conditions for violence—what Michelle Murphy (2013, 2) refers to as "the spatially and temporally extensive ways that practices are sedimented into and structure the world"—is a counter to the politics of potential. As Murphy explains, "A capacious sense of infrastructures includes social sedimentations such as colonial legacies, the repetition of gendered norms in material culture, or the persistence of racialization" (2). In South Africa, the legacies of settler colonialism and apartheid for migration patterns, family structures, and high rates of interpersonal violence produce gendered infrastructures of anticipation that have profound effects on intergenerational relations. The first 1,000 days image of futurity concentrates on the figure of the mother as agential environment, but does not recognize the historical and social factors that structure the relations that make for the uneven distribution of potential futures.

CONCLUSION
The Politics of Potential

My ethnographic findings show how global health policy and practice is shaped by a politics of potential that has three key tenets. First, that the substance of potential is found only in specific people and places and not in others. Second, that the manifesting of potential is an action of individual responsibility, rather than of collective or structural forces. Third, that potential is understood from the perspective of an already given future end and not from the perspective of the durative present. Such a politics excludes other social actors from view, obscures a need for collective responsibility toward historical injury, and overlooks the potentialities that structure life in the present.

THE SUBSTANCE OF POTENTIAL

Actions or interventions designed to augment potential foreground specific groups and overlook others. The first 1,000 days powerfully articulates a politics of potential that prioritizes investment in early life interventions and predominantly targets female bodies as the protectors of future human capital. The mother and child are central figures in the stylized images of the first 1,000 days and as key targets of clinical interventions. The politics of potential thus dictates inclusion or exclusion from a therapeutic citizenship—a political subjectivity that permits resource claims from the state and other agencies on the basis of biological categories (Nguyen 2005). This therapeutic citizenship is predicated on forms of intimacy perceived as worthy of state and global concern. In this sense, it extends a colonial logic that sought to inculcate a notion of motherhood as an individual project—what some have termed "intimate colonialism" (Summers 1991, 787). The biological subject of global health takes on a strange dual role in interventions such as the first 1,000 days: the mother-child dyad is both the universal, globalized body of the development agenda, amenable to large-scale interventions across continents for the sake of humanity and the future, and also an entity whose power lies in its plasticity.

Fathers and young men do not feature prominently in this configuration, if they figure at all. There is a subtle exclusion of men and young boys from the public health gaze and from social concern that reflects the "reproductive grammar" of the state (Franklin and Ginsburg 2019, 4). As James Ferguson (2015, 40) has suggested, traditional welfare recipients (including "the child" and "the dependent reproductive woman") constitute "a kind of photographic negative of the figure of the wage-earning man." In the context of very high rates of unemployment, men in South Africa have lost the "full public citizenship" that work affords, while children and their (female) caregivers retain a form of citizenship through their recognition as "dependent" on the state. As Elena Moore and Jeremy Seekings (2019, 518) state, "through both providing grants to some individuals within households and families and denying them to others, the state has recast relations of dependency within households and families as much as between its citizens and the state itself."

Although the state in South Africa is often dysfunctional, it remains an important mediator in assemblages of global health. Beyond the provision of health care, the state is a central facilitator of the future-making projects of citizens through the established welfare system of social grants, state provision of housing, and other benefits. Even though my interlocutors complained about the difficulties of obtaining a grant or a title deed or sending a child to a preferred school, they had not given up on navigating the state as a provider of the resources that would help them build a desired future. They fully expected that such state provisions should continue and that "one day they would make it right." I concur with James Ferguson (2015), who draws on a parent-child metaphor to understand the strong sense among South Africans that the state has social obligations to care for all its citizens. Yet it is (female) caregivers who were largely the recipients of state welfare until the introduction of COVID-19 relief grants in 2020. If "intimate colonialism" was about the import of imperial projects of motherhood, women are still granted a form of recognition, or intimate citizenship, by virtue of their capacity to perform reproductive work. Women thus craft gendered political subjectivities via reproductive and domestic labor in ways that are unavailable to men. As Sophie Oldfield and colleagues (2019, 47) argue, "negotiations for citizenship start with women's bodies and are forged in the private sphere in homes." For young unemployed men in Cape Town, dignity and belonging is sometimes tragically sought via other routes that include gang membership (Jensen 2008). In sum, despite some efforts to expand the state's recognition of kinship beyond biological relations in the provision of social welfare in South Africa, there are distinctly gendered continuities in how subjects are enfolded into or excluded from biomedical regimes and projects of citizenship.

There are also distinct continuities between the DOHaD focus on "transitioning societies" and historical interventions in "the developing world." Why do some places and people fall under the gaze of DOHaD while others do not? The international DOHaD conference held in Cape Town illustrated how scientists, clinicians, and public health experts translate the language of DOHaD and epigenetics into applied policy with a sharp focus on "transitioning societies." The northern scientist's quip that the DOHaD brain is in the North and its nether regions in the South points to the persistence of older knowledge hierarchies, even though much DOHaD research is produced by scientists based in Asia and Africa. With his assertion that Africa is "the omphalos—the source of nourishment," the DOHaD scientist reinvented Africa again (Mudimbé 1988) as a place of discovery and as a site for extraction and intervention.

Just as knowledge production around global health has been influenced by a dominant set of temporal and spatial logics around globalization, postgenomic research has produced DOHaD geographies (Pentecost 2018b). DOHaD research is especially concerned with regions often glossed as the Global South, which researchers characterize as burdened by the dual public health burdens of child undernutrition and adult obesity, based on the understanding that these regions are undergoing nutrition transition (Popkin et al. 2011). Yet demographers and social scientists have questioned the usefulness of transition theories (Frenk et al. 1989; Chen et al. 1993; Ulijaszek et al. 2012). They argue that transitions are not linear or universal: patterns overlap and local, historical, and political-economic factors account for unique configurations of transition. Despite this extensive scrutiny, the concept of "transitioning societies" remains prominent in public health models (Yates-Doerr 2015a). The idea that "transitioning societies" demarcate geographical regions of concern for DOHaD science may suggest the unreflexive application of transition theory (Carolina and Gustavo 2003) or it may point to a persistent attachment to transition narratives (Chakrabarty 1992) that recreate subtle divisions of power that have continuities with the colonial and development eras. As I have argued throughout, careful attention is required to track how new understandings of heredity shape policy under the rubric of global health, especially where the antecedents of such policies lie in development projects and colonial intervention.

THE MANIFESTING OF POTENTIAL

A politics of potential configures individuals as agents who are responsible for future outcomes regardless of their present material circumstances. Perinatal nutrition policy and its implementation hinges on individual responsibility and compliance even in the face of chronic food insecurity and dysfunctional health systems. This logic is most apparent in the Nutrition Therapeutic Program's exit codes—"successful," "unsuccessful," "interrupted"—which make no allowance for the structural factors that militate against a patient successfully completing the program and do not include a requirement that clinic staff ask about the circumstances that have warranted supplementation. Such a framing elides the reality of chronic hunger.

As accounts throughout this book make clear, many families subsist on meager incomes cobbled together from a variety of sources that are subject to seasonal fluctuations and claims from kin and creditors. As Sindi explained, the problem is not that women do not know what a healthy diet looks like; the problem is that healthy food is not available or affordable. A focus on individual responsibility overlooks the obstacles of physical distance from food outlets that stock healthier options, the expense of travel outside the township, and the price of a diverse diet. For many, a diet of low dietary diversity is the norm. Others are almost entirely reliant on the food supplements they might receive from the clinic—which are not supplements at all, but a substitute for daily sustenance.

Although hunger relief is a central focus of humanitarian interventions elsewhere, hunger in Khayelitsha's clinics was easily "unknown," looked over in the performative completion of registers and audits and in the boundaries staff drew for themselves with the statement that "there's nothing I can do." The blurring of the lines between "pharmaceutical," "food," and "supplement" and "patient," "consumer," and "citizen" re-inscribes responsibility and redistributes the concern for ethical action in the present. Ready-to-use therapeutic foods in this context are not emergency palliatives to secure present survival. Rather, they are state-delivered reproductive technologies that are meant to shape the future.

THE FRAMING OF POTENTIAL

Closely linked to the question of "how societies produce and reproduce themselves" is how societies conceive of the future (Munn 1992). Jane Guyer's seminal work (2007) argues that the "near future" is in decline as a temporal frame in public and theoretical representations. She describes a shift toward "both very short and very long sightedness, with a symmetrical evacuation of the near past and the near future" (410). Guyer surmises that life is increasingly governed by "date regimes" in which "the world itself falls increasingly into the disciplines of a punctuated time that fills the gap between an instantaneous present and an altogether different distant future" (417). The first 1,000 days is one such date regime, and in this book I have sought to describe the futures that ethnography might find between the immediate horizon and the very distant horizons that seem to dominate forms and representations.

Some futures are more valid than others. This was evident in the different futures that were articulated in the various sites of this study, from the performance of the future in policy discourse, to the aspirations and setbacks of my interlocutors, to the ways the future conditions experiences of the present. My attention to the future in the context of Khayelitsha, both in the representational sense and the affective sense, revealed the important disjunctures between the temporal orientations of the first 1,000 days and the everyday ways that anticipation structures action. All of my participants desired "the best" for their children—the happy future that the first 1,000 days campaign conjures. However, in contrast to the policy focus on individual agency, the construction of futures in Khayelitsha was predicated on the ability to navigate opportunities accessible through the state, NGOs, one's own networks, and the reciprocities and debts that accompanied each of these. Hopeful visions of the future, which were often reflected in an infant's name, were confronted with bureaucratic time, with the economic time of credits and debts, with God's time, and for some, like Songezwa and Sithembele, with the sense that time had run out. The most searing distortion of time and the future, however, was wrought by the constant potential for violence. Life was lived in a different register of anticipation. The always-existing potential for violence produced a structure of anticipation that configured the ordinary movements of people I met as they went to work, took their children to school, shopped for groceries, attended the clinic, worshiped at church, and visited friends or relatives. This structuring force extended even to reproductive desires, reflected in an ambivalence during pregnancy about the challenges of rearing sons.

The first 1,000 days concept includes a teleological view that action in the present will be judged at some point in the future and that this ethical judgement extends across future generations. As Elizabeth Povinelli (2011) argues, teleological discourses that assume an already given end allow for a reading of ethics "from the perspective of future ends. . . . The ethical nature of present action is interpreted from the point of view of a reflexive future horizon" (3). In opposition to this stands the durative present, in which the ethical nature of present action can be interpreted only in the context of the present moment. Actions in the present are not configured by some distant actualization of potential but by potentialities that are always already existing and persistent. Here, potential is not the precursor to what will certainly be actualized in the classic Aristotelian sense. Rather, potential persists regardless of whether it is actualized or not. In the case of violence, even if the event does not arrive, its anticipation is a constant force that structures life and affect (see Das 2007). As Pumla Dineo Gqola (2021) notes, fear is a language, and fluency is expected of women. Potentialities that are rooted in postcolonial, racist, and heteropatriarchal violence structure action in the present and are elided in frameworks that defer an ethical reading of action to some distant future point.

Alongside the politics of potential is the politics of trauma. A question arises as to how to apprehend the effects of violence in the context of revised understandings of heredity. I suggest that the discourse of trauma, which is readily deployed in both academic and popular arenas in South Africa to explain cyclical patterns of violence, is ill suited to this task. The possibility of "epigenetic trauma" is discussed in DOHaD and epigenetic studies to describe a host of intergenerational exposures, including war, slavery, famine, and racism (Jasienska 2009; Kuzawa and Sweet 2009; Yehuda and Lehrner 2018). As Michel Dubois and Catherine Guaspare (2020, 153) have argued, "epigenetic trauma" becomes a descriptor that encompasses a broad range of "traumatic pasts" in "very different periods and places." Although some groups mobilize a discourse of social epigenetics for social justice, such as Indigenous communities in Australia (Kowal and Warin 2018), a framework of epigenetic trauma imposed from outside risks new forms of reductionism and narratives of "damage" (Tuck 2009) that foreground harm instead of reversibility (Meloni and Müller 2018). In South Africa, the mobilization of the notion that trauma is transmitted from generation to generation epigenetically as an explanation for patterns of violence is a dangerous biologized view of the bodily manifestations of apartheid history. It is itself a reinscription of damage and a form of violence.

Applying a framework of trauma in this case falsely identifies crisis as the exception, when in fact crisis is ordinary (Berlant 2011). A traumatic structure, as Nancy Rose Hunt has argued in her analysis of colonial Belgian Congo (2016), conforms to a linear narrative of before and after, event and aftermath, and cause and effect that passes over plasticity, uncertainty, and the ordinary. It focuses on the spectacular while overlooking what is not amenable to the forms of aggregation and evaluation that political recognition requires: what Elizabeth Povinelli terms quasi-events.

Quasi-events "never quite achieve the status of having occurred or taken place. They neither happen nor not happen" (Povinelli 2011, 13). The quasi-event is the daily encounter with a bullet hole in the refrigerator. It is the quiet binge of the methamphetamine addict between household mealtimes. It is the hiding of a cereal box under the bed so there will be breakfast for the children before school. It is offering food to a child who will not sleep despite the repeated whispers of "Akukho nto izakwenzeka'" ("Nothing will happen").

Quasi-events are not perceptible in epigenetic and DOHaD understandings of the "environment." Just as these scientific discourses atomize the maternal body as their unit of intervention, a discourse of trauma reduces the possibilities for intervention to what is perceptible in epidemiological terms.

HIDDEN POTENTIAL

This sketch of a politics of potential as one framework for understanding the first 1,000 days concept—and thus new formations of postgenomic knowledge, global health, and the future—is, like all theories, a simplification that captures key elements for their possible application elsewhere. At the same time I have also followed those stories that do not allow for closed endings but rather reveal other hidden potential: what I have termed life between protocols. Take Nobomi's tactical use of clinical trials, for example, or Sr. Qoma's selective interpretation of the infant feeding policy to allocate available resources to those most in need. What of the nursing sister who deviates from the standardized performance of care—forgetting to ask a patient to remove her jacket before her weight is measured or omitting a MUAC reading because the patient is visibly obese? Or consider again how Inam dutifully takes supplements home, where the peanut butter sachets and milkshakes are consumed by the children rather than by Inam herself. These examples all point to life between protocols: moments configured by wit, cunning, care, or apathy that constitute these scenes of relating.

At a different scale, writing "life between" contributes to efforts in urban scholarship to write the South African city outside obvious frameworks of segregation and inequality (Nuttall and Mbembe 2008; Simone 2004; Le Marcis 2004; Gillespie 2015) of which depictions of Khayelitsha have been especially prone. Comaroff and Comaroff (2016, 190) describe Khayelitsha as "effectively vacated by the state." This offers a tempting analysis for understanding my observations. Yet while my ethnographic findings underscore the powerful effects of the potential for violence in structuring how life is lived in Khayelitsha, I disagree that "criminality has become *the* constitutive fact of contemporary life, *the* vernacular in terms of which politics is conducted, moral panics are voiced, [and] populations are ruled" (xiii, emphasis in original). The making and unmaking of futures is heavily influenced by the presence of violence *and* by other frames that include the state and its bureaucracies, the market, nostalgia, and religion. A methodological question thus arises about what kinds of evidence produce what kinds of analyses; ethnography close to the ground tends to counter any easy foreclosures.

Writing "life between" is also a way to refute linear knowledge flows. South African science has played a key role in DOHaD research, disrupting any simple North-South categorizations of scientific knowledge production in this field. This book might be described as a policy ethnography or an ethnography of the place of South Africa in global health, but it is also an ethnography of everyday life in Khayelitsha in post-apartheid Cape Town. Khayelitsha is at once a "truth spot" (Herrick 2017, 530) for the production of global health knowledge and a site that reveals the tensions and contradictions of global health campaigns that overlook dynamic urban life and kinship. Pushing against the common juxtaposition of city and township, Khayelitsha is better understood as a node in a much wider set of networks that might be indexed by clinical trials, rural-urban circulations, supermarket chains, nongovernmental organizations, research teams, charismatic churches, international conferences, savings groups, or allocations of police resources. At the same time, my interlocutors' struggles with the high risk of crime where they live, securing a place in a decent school, or attending a hospital where they feel cared for are part of the difficult realities of being resident in this part of the city. Rather than repeating an image of the township and its problems as separate (Gillespie 2014), I have attempted in this book to articulate the set of "body-city configurations" (Solomon 2016, 15) that move into focus with a decentered view, and have demonstrated how these are profoundly gendered (see also McKay 2018b). Integrating a biosocial framework, I extend this frame further: I argue that a thorough analysis of how forms and effects of global health manifest can put neither people nor places first (Biehl and Petryna 2013; Herrick 2017; Neely and Nading 2017) but must offer deep and sustained attention to how bodies and environments are made and remade together over time in particular sociopolitical milieus.

THE EXPANDING CATEGORY OF EARLY LIFE

In 2016, the Western Cape provincial government expanded its focus on the first 1,000 days beyond nutrition policy with the First 1000 Days: Right Start, Bright Future campaign (Western Cape Government First 1000 Days Campaign 2016), which was jointly run by the Department of Health and the Department of Social Development. The campaign's motto—"Grow, love, play"—referred to a triad of recommendations for good nutrition, maternal attention, and play and stimulation. This expansion of the first 1,000 days concept includes forms of care, play, and even love as desirable policy outcomes based on research in biology and developmental psychology that links interactions between genes and environment, parental investment, neurodevelopment, and self-regulation (Pentecost and Ross 2019).

The DOHaD evidence base has also expanded from observational to intervention studies and the focus has shifted to the timing of interventions. More recent findings from intervention trials during pregnancy have shown limited evidence of efficacy (Heslehurst et al. 2019), and there is increased interest in interventions prior to conception to shape intergenerational health (Stephenson et al. 2018). The category of "early life" has now come to encompass childhood, infancy, pregnancy, and preconception—a period that is vaguely defined and potentially includes all adults of reproductive age (Pentecost and Meloni 2020).

It remains to be seen whether social context might be understood and accounted for in preconception interventions, given the possibilities they have to amplify or diminish attention to the social drivers of health inequities. As I and others have argued, early life interventions focused on pregnancy have produced a highly gendered discourse of responsibility for health outcomes. The expansion of the notion of early life to include the preconception period as a target of intervention has the potential for the further gendered allocation of responsibility and the biomedicalization of female bodies. The utility of the preconception frame will hinge on whether it can reflect a broader set of social concerns that do not center on women of reproductive age in isolation or as the target of individual interventions but instead encompass structural determinants of health and center justice and equity.

In the regimes of recognition that such framings afford, will the dyad remain at the center of interventions? Will epigenetic responsibility (Hedlund 2011) remain firmly on the shoulders of the liberal (maternal) subject? What might be obscured in the registers of transmission, trauma, and resilience that seem ready at hand? As the definition of early life expands and formalizes new categories for intervention, close attention will be needed to how concepts of health, heredity, and development produce new forms of governmentality and manifest material, ethical, and social concerns. All indicators point to the persistence of a politics of potential that foregrounds women of reproductive age as the responsible arbiters of health and the future.

ACKNOWLEDGMENTS

This research was primarily funded by the Commonwealth Scholarship Commission in the United Kingdom and I thank the commission for making this project financially possible. I also received assistance from the School of Anthropology & Museum Ethnography at the University of Oxford; Green Templeton College, University of Oxford; the Medical and Health Humanities Africa network; the National Science Foundation; the Andrew W. Mellon Foundation as part of Fiona Ross's First Thousand Days Research Group; and the King's College London Social Science and Public Policy Publication Subvention Fund.

This book would not have been possible without the generosity and support of many people. In Cape Town, I owe a huge debt of gratitude to the research participants and my research assistant, although I cannot identify them by name here. My research assistant, who was also a close interlocutor, was indispensable to this project. I extend my utmost gratitude to her for her companionship during fieldwork and for her participation in this research. Women and their families gave generously of their time during their pregnancies and the first months of their children's lives—it was a privilege to share that time with them. I extend my heartfelt thanks to the government staff, clinic staff, scientists, clinicians, and policymakers who participated in this project. During fieldwork in Cape Town, I benefited from the insights and support of Yashar Taheri-Keramati, Erin Torkelson, Nontsasa Nyovane, Nosiphiwo Gwadiso, Shariefa-Patel Abrahams, Hilary Goeiman, Virginia Adriaans, and Edna Arends. I am also grateful for the formative conversations and encouragement of Lesley Bourne, Mark Tomlinson, David Sanders, Steve Reid, Janet Giddy, Dinky Levitt, and Katherine Everett Murphy. I learned isiXhosa during fieldwork with the help of Xhosa Fundis.

I owe a debt of gratitude to the mentors who have helped me navigate the path of physician-anthropologist over the years. I am grateful to Steve Reid, Susan Levine, Marc Blockman, and Paul Roux, who supported my unusual decision, in the South African context, to pursue a doctorate in anthropology following my medical degree. I thank Stanley Ulijaszek for his unwavering support of this project from the start and for his stewardship, grace, and patience. I thank Fiona Ross for her generous mentorship and for our close collaboration over the last decade, which has indelibly shaped this work. This book would not have been completed without her nourishing friendship and encouragement. Vinh-Kim Nguyen is a mentor in the true sense of the word—a wise and trusted counselor. I cannot thank him enough for what he has taught me about how to be a doctor, a scholar, a teacher, and a friend.

This research has multiple institutional homes. At the University of Oxford, I found a vibrant scholarly community. I am grateful for the teaching and guidance of Alex Alvergne, Morgan Clarke, Elizabeth Ewart, David Gellner, Javier Lezaun, Caroline Potter, David Pratten, Ramon Sarró, and Alison Shaw. I thank Vicky Dean, Elizabeth Iles, Kate Atherton, and Michelle Mhlanga for their support. The Unit for Biocultural Variation and Obesity at the University of Oxford provided space for critical thought and collegiality; I thank Stanley Ulijaszek for his leadership and the UBVO community for our many enriching conversations. I found camaraderie and inspiration during my studies with my peers Marthe Achtnich, Maan Barua, Julia Binter, Tess Bird, Alex Budzier, Anna Custers, Casper Thomas, Hannah Dawson, Adam Gilbertson, Jenny Hough, Nadine Levin, Amy McLennan, Seonsam Na, Steph Postar, Cory Rodgers, Kate Roll, Laurel Steinfeld, Darryl Stellmach, Morten Hansen, and Astrid van den Bossche. I thank Stanley Ulijaszek, Pauline Ulijaszek, Alex Alvergne, Morgan Clarke, David Gellner, Lola Martinez, Jonny Steinberg, Lomin Saayman, Jocelyn Alexander, Deborah James, Patrick Pearson, Jamie Lorimer, Magali Tang, Ann Kelly, and Javier Lezaun for their friendship and generosity.

At the University of Cape Town, Fiona Ross created an exciting space of inquiry in The First Thousand Days Research Group. Many thanks to Kate Abney, Deidre Blackie, Nicole Ferreira, Kathleen McDougall, Tessa Moll, Min'enhle Ncube, Efua Prah, Yusra Price, Jennifer Rogerson, Nanna Schneidermann, Carina Truyts, Miriam Waltz, Anusha Lachman, and Astrid Berg for the fruitful collaborations and friendships that emerged from that group. I also thank Pamela Reynolds, whose pioneering work on the anthropology of early life in southern Africa has been so formative for this project.

This work took shape alongside the exciting development of the Medical and Health Humanities Africa network. Many thanks to Steve Reid, Susan Levine, Catherine Burns, Nolwazi Mkhwanazi, Carla Tsampiras, Victoria Hume, Berna Gerber, Megan Wainwright, Guddi Singh, Ferdinand Mukumbang, Lizahn Cloete, Chris Colvin, Hayley MacGregor, Leslie Swartz, Thomas Cousins, and the MHHA community for formative conversations, gatherings, and collaborations over the past ten years.

I completed this manuscript in the company of excellent colleagues at the Department of Global Health & Social Medicine at King's College London. Heartfelt thanks to all of my colleagues, especially to Bronwyn Parry, Nikolas Rose, Ann Kelly, and Anne Pollock for their unwavering encouragement and to Carlo Caduff and the members of the Culture, Medicine & Power research group for feedback on drafts of the manuscript. Final revisions were possible due to the generosity of colleagues at the Graduate Institute in Geneva during my visits there, and I am indebted to Vinh-Kim Nguyen for helping me create the time and space needed to see this project through to completion.

I benefited from the feedback of several audiences and conversations at annual meetings and conferences: in 2015, the Johannesburg Workshop for Theory and Criticism and the Anthropology Southern Africa conference; in 2016, the Association of Social Anthropologists of the UK and Commonwealth and a gathering at the Brocher Foundation; and in 2019, the annual meeting of the American Anthropological Association. I also attended the University College London Medical Anthropology seminar, several conferences of the Society for the Social Studies of Science, and gatherings at the Wits Institute for Social and Economic Research, the Stellenbosch Institute for Advanced Studies, and the anthropology departments at the University of Oxford and the University of Cape Town. At these and other meetings I was grateful for the generous engagement of colleagues, including Megan Vaughan, Julie Livingston, Catherine Burns, Nolwazi Mkhwanazi, Lenore Manderson, Kaushik Sunder-Rajan, Noah Tamarkin, Eileen Moyer, Susan Levine, Ilana van Wyk, Rose Marie Beck, Abdallah Daar, Birgit Meyer, Joseph Tonda, Andrew Macnab, Hayley MacGregor, Todd Meyers, Danya Glabau, Lucy Lowe, Ian Harper, Maya Unnithan, Marina Marouda, Margaret Sleeboom-Faulkner, Maurizio Meloni, Tatjana Buklijas, Megan Warin, Martyn Pickersgill, Ramah McKay, Sahra Gibbon, Janelle Lamoreaux, Elizabeth Roberts, Stephanie Lloyd, Amber Benezra, Martine Lappé, Robin Jeffries-Hein, Katie Dow, Michi Penkler, Emily Yates-Doerr, Natali Valdez, Edna Bosire, Andrew Kim, Emily Mendenhall, Eugene Raikhel, and Vincanne Adams.

Excerpts of this book appear in collaborative publications elsewhere. Chapter 3 includes excerpts from "The First 1000 Days: Epigenetics in the Age of Global Health," a chapter in the *Palgrave Handbook of Biology and Society*, edited by Maurizio Meloni, John Cromby, Des Fitzgerald, and Stephanie Lloyd (Palgrave Macmillan, 2018). Chapter 6 includes excerpts from "The Politics of Trauma: Gender, Futurity and Violence Prevention in South Africa," published in a 2022 special issue of *Medical Anthropology Quarterly* titled "Toward Intergenerational Ethnography: Kinship, Cohorts, and Environments in and Beyond the Biosocial Sciences," edited by Sahra Gibbon and Janelle Lamoreaux.

The editorial stewardship of Lenore Manderson and Kimberly Guinta has been invaluable in helping me realize this project. I owe a debt of gratitude to Lenore for her keen editorial eye and her encouragement and enthusiasm and to Kimberly for her close attention to this work. I also extend thanks to Kathleen Kelly, Eliza Cubitt and Kate Babbitt for their editorial input and to Miles Irving for the maps that appear in this book. I am grateful to Vincent Bezuidenhout for permission to feature his aerial photograph *False Bay #1* and for the important ways his work shaped my thoughts on perspective during this research. I am also honored to feature the work *Siwum'ndeni (We are family)* of artist Zanele Montle on the cover.

I extend a special thanks to my family, especially my parents Brian and Patricia Pentecost and to my grandmother Hilma Moodie for their unfailing love. Many thanks also to Ben Cousins, Anne Saunderson-Meyer, and Colleen Crawford-Cousins for their support. I am also forever indebted to Jocelyn Hellig for always being my home away from home.

This work is dedicated to Thomas. It owes much to his constant love and encouragement.

NOTES

INTRODUCTION

1. A township in the South African context refers (usually) to an urban residential area historically reserved for people classified as "African," "Coloured," or "Indian" who worked or lived near "White only" areas under apartheid segregation laws.

2. Throughout the text, non-English words are not italicized except for emphasis. The intention is to refuse stylistic structures that designate foreignness and to insist on a story told from multiple vantage points that does not reproduce assumptions about audience and subject (see Ha 2018; Verissimo 2019; Cousins 2023).

3. The use of racial categories in this text does not imply an acceptance of racial attributes of any sort. Their use references the violent history of racial classification in colonial and apartheid South Africa and contemporary state classifications that are the subject of intense debate (Posel 2001; Erasmus 2008; Dubow 2014). The Population Registration Act of 1950, a key piece of legislation underpinning "high apartheid" (Dubow 2017), decreed that each person should carry an identity document that recorded their race as either "White," "Coloured," or "Native"; this was later modified to divide the population into four groups: "African," "Indian" "Coloured," and "White" (Posel 2001). In democratic South Africa, the national census categorizes persons as "Black African," "White," "Coloured," or "Indian/Asian." The use of these categories as per the census throughout the text serves to historicize these terms and to dislodge the residual essentialism that the terms black or white might imply. See also Appiah 2020 on the capitalization of "Black" and "White."

4. The construction of the concept of the "environment" has been a key question for social studies of DOHaD and epigenetic science (see Landecker 2011; Lock and Palsson 2016; Shostak and Moinester 2015; Lamoreaux 2016; Valdez 2021; and Penkler 2022).

5. This third premise follows Elizabeth Povinelli's (2011) understanding of tense and the judgment of ethical action.

6. See Robins (2004) for an overview of the complex terrain of the cultural politics of HIV in South Africa in the 2000s.

7. There is a significant social science literature on HIV in South Africa; some key texts include Robins (2004), Fassin (2007), Nattrass (2008), Fassin (2015), and Cousins (2016).

8. The hiring of research assistants for conducting fieldwork brings its own ethical challenges and the need for awareness of how the research may be shaped by the triangulation of power relations between researcher, assistant, and participant (Deane and Stevano 2016). Nomsa's background was very similar to that of many of the women we worked with. She was in her late 20s when this study was conducted and was living with her husband and child in Khayelitsha. She had completed secondary school and was working toward a diploma to enhance her chances of finding work in administration. As an assistant, she helped keep records of participants' contact details (which would frequently change) and used her clear understanding of local conditions in Khayelitsha to help us navigate the township as safely as possible. With training, she took her own ethnographic notes on our field visits; along with her local knowledge, these helped corroborate and add to my observations in our daily reflective conversations. While writing this monograph was a single-author endeavor, a model to which anthropology as a discipline remains curiously wed, Nomsa's assistance during fieldwork was

indispensable and her story as both research assistant and research participant is inextricably woven throughout these pages.

9. The concept of the clinic has received robust treatment by medical anthropologists. For key texts, see Chatterji et al. (1998), Das and Das (2006), Goodfellow (2014), Carney (2015), and Meyers (2013).

10. Pseudonyms have been used.

11. Names of interlocutors, clinics, and clinic staff have been changed to protect confidentiality.

12. For a detailed discussion of the construction of "community" in global health initiatives see McKay (2018a).

13. See, for example, the 2006 special issue of *American Anthropologist* co-edited by Frances E. Mascia-Lees and Patricia Sharpe, Didier Fassin and colleagues' use of *Life and Times of Michael K* (2008), Pamela Reynolds's use of boyhood in *War in Worcester* (2013), and Veena Das's (2006) discussions of Coetzee, in dialogue with Wittgenstein, concerning "violence, authority, and the authoritative voice."

CHAPTER 1   THE FIRST 1,000 DAYS

1. For work in biological anthropology, see Benyshek et al. (2001), Benyshek (2007), Kuzawa and Sweet (2009), Thayer and Kuzawa (2011), and Goodman (2013). For new frameworks in medical anthropology, see Margaret Lock's "local biologies" (2013, 1993), Jorg Niewöhner's "embedded bodies" (2011), Tim Ingold and Gisli Palsson's "biosocial becomings" (2013), and Megan Warin and colleagues' "biohabitus" (2015).

2. For key social science texts on epigenetics, see Pickersgill et al. (2013) and Meloni and Testa (2014). For texts on the figure of the maternal body in epigenetic science, see Richardson (2015), Warin (2012), Mansfield (2012), Kenney and Müller (2017), Pentecost and Ross (2019), and Valdez (2021).

3. Also described as fetal impression (Paneth 1994), genomic imprinting (Signorello and Trichopoulos 1998), metabolic imprinting (Waterland and Garza 1999), and induction (Bateson 2001).

4. The Alma-Ata Declaration was the outcome of an international primary health care conference in September 1978 in what is now Kazakhstan, where participating countries adopted the primary health care approach as the key to achieving "Health for All."

5. UNICEF, formed in 1946 by the UN General Assembly, stands for the United Nations International Children's Emergency Fund. It is known today as the United Nations Children's Fund.

6. The Millennium Development Goals were (1) the eradication of extreme poverty and hunger, (2) provision of universal primary education, (3) promotion of gender equality, (4) reduction of child mortality, (5) improvement of maternal health, (6) a focus on HIV/AIDS and malaria, (7) promotion of environmental sustainability, and (8) creation of a global partnership for development (UN 2000).

7. 1,000 Days is a US-based advocacy group partnered with the US Department of State, the UN's Scaling Up Nutrition movement, the Global Alliance for Improved Nutrition, and the Bill & Melinda Gates Foundation, among others (see thousanddays.org).

8. Natal is now KwaZulu-Natal.

9. For detailed histories of this period, see Posel (1991), Beinart and Dubow (1995), and Dubow (2014).

10. The apartheid government declared that bantustan territories were independent homelands. Those opposed to apartheid rejected the term "homeland" because it obscured the

exclusionary nature of these divisions. They preferred the word "bantustan," in order to signal the "artificiality of configuring geographical regions so as to correspond to supposed 'tribal' divisions" (Beinart and Dubow 1995, 16).

11. The South African Demographic and Health Survey of 2007, the National Income Dynamics Study of 2009 (Ardington and Case 2009), and the South African Health and Nutrition Survey of 2013 (Shisana et al. 2013).

12. See, for example, Vorster et al. (1999), Bourne et al. (2002), and Steyn et al. (2012).

13. Integrated Regional Information Networks (IRIN) News was founded by the United Nations in 1995. In 2019, the name changed. This news is now published on the UN's The New Humanitarian website.

14. For a comprehensive overview of infant feeding policy in South Africa from 1980 to 2018, see Nieuwoudt et al. (2019).

CHAPTER 2   SITUATED BIOLOGIES

1. During apartheid, Mitchell's Plain was reserved for people designated as Coloured.

2. In 2014, the City of Cape Town underwent a controversial rebranding exercise of its corporate identity. Mayor Patricia de Lille announced that the city's new slogan was "Making Progress Possible. Together," which was intended to avoid implying a "passive government-citizen relationship" (De Lille 2014).

3. The food poverty line refers to the amount of money an individual needs to consume enough food to maintain an average energy level, as devised by Statistics South Africa based on the Statistics Division of the United Nations (Statistics South Africa 2008).

4. R6,500 was approximately US$600 at the time of the 2011 census.

5. The Gini coefficient is a statistical measure of income inequality.

6. A syndemic refers to the coexistence and adverse interaction of multiple health conditions that manifest in contexts of socioeconomic inequality and produce stress and material deprivation; see Singer et al. (2017) for a full account of syndemic theory.

7. Food insecurity refers to the sustained lack of physical and economic access to enough safe and nutritious foods to meet dietary needs and accommodate food preferences.

CHAPTER 3   THE TRAVELING TECHNOLOGY OF MOTHER AND CHILD

1. See Yates-Doerr (2015b) for further discussion of the problems of scaling as a global health technology.

2. "Matric" refers to the end of secondary school.

3. See Manderson and Ross (2020) for a full overview.

4. Nursing staff (female and male) are called "sister" in the South African medical system.

5. About US$38 at that time.

6. About US$82 at that time, well below what would be considered a minimum wage.

7. Registrars are doctors undergoing specialty training in the South African medical system; Public Health is a specialty focused on epidemiology and community health.

CHAPTER 4   LIFE BETWEEN PROTOCOLS

1. A health promoter's role is to offer patient education, often in the form of group lectures, group discussions or individual counselling.

2. Bactrim is the brand name of an antibiotic given routinely to infants exposed to or infected by HIV to prevent *Pneumocystis jiroveci* pneumonia, a frequent opportunistic infection in the context of HIV.

3. The acronym AFASS—for acceptable, feasible, affordable, sustainable, and safe—first appeared in recommendations on HIV and infant feeding in 2007. It was designed to assist in assessing whether formula feeding was an appropriate choice for an infant, given that formula feeding requires adequate water and sanitation and the means to prepare and store milk (World Health Organization 2007).

4. The CD4 count is a lab measurement of the number of CD4 T lymphocytes and is used as a marker of immune function and disease progression in HIV infection. Historically it was used to determine when antiretroviral therapy should be initiated. From January 2015, all HIV-positive pregnant and breastfeeding women were initiated on lifelong antiretroviral therapy regardless of CD4 count at their first appointment at a clinic (Burton et al. 2015).

5. The MUAC metric has been incorporated into South Africa's Maternity Case Record document as a simpler measure of nutritional status because height does not have to checked, no calculations are required, and unlike weight, MUAC is fairly constant throughout pregnancy (Department of Health, Republic of South Africa 2015).

6. See Hansen et al. (2015) for a comprehensive guide to the criteria for entering the Nutrition Therapeutic Program and the products specified for each target group.

7. The honorific "sister" was originally used for nuns undertaking nursing as part of their religious duties. Now both female and male nurses are called "sister" in South Africa, despite the implication that nursing is feminine labor (Kalemba 2020).

8. Approximately US$24 at that time.

9. A main road in Khayelitsha connected to the N2 highway.

CHAPTER 5   INTERGENERATIONAL TRANSMISSIONS

1. Approximately US$95 at that time.

2. A suburb in Khayelitsha with the highest house prices in the township.

3. Somerset West is an affluent suburb around the Helderberg Mountains, east of Khayelitsha.

4. Constantia is a high-income suburb in central Cape Town.

5. Soweto is the largest township in Gauteng Province; Clifton and Umhlanga Rocks are affluent seaside towns in Cape Town and Durban, respectively.

6. According to Bathandwa's husband, a house in Khayelitsha would have cost US$800 dollars in 2001 and US$9,000 in 2015. In Ilitha Park, a house would have sold for US$45,000 in 2015. In 2022, a house in that neighborhood would sell for US$67,000.

7. Standard Six is the first year of secondary school; Grade Twelve is the last year.

8. See Kalumba (2017) for a dictionary of South African names and their meanings.

9. June 16, 1976, was the day of the Soweto uprising, a mass youth-led protest against the addition of Afrikaans as a medium of instruction in schools. The apartheid police killed hundreds of protestors, many of them children. In 1994, June 16 was declared a public holiday (Youth Day) in remembrance of this event.

10. A title deed is a legal document that proves ownership of property.

11. Approximately US$1,600.

12. This accords with anthropologist Kelly Gillespie's reports to the Khayelitsha Commission, which stated that the taxi associations "run a formidable alternative justice system" (quoted in Khayelitsha Commission 2014, 139).

REFERENCES

Adams, Vincanne. 2016. *Metrics: What Counts in Global Health*. Durham, NC: Duke University Press.

Adams, Vincanne, Michelle Murphy, and Adele E. Clarke. 2009. "Anticipation: Technoscience, Life, Affect, Temporality." *Subjectivity* 28: 246–265. https://doi.org/10.1057/sub.2009.18.

Adonis, Cyril K. 2016. "Exploring the Salience of Intergenerational Trauma among Children and Grandchildren of Victims of Apartheid-era Gross Human Rights Violations," *Indo-Pacific Journal of Phenomenology* 16:163–79.

Affordable Land & Housing Data Centre. 2013. "Suburb Profiles: Khayelitsha." Accessed June 1, 2014. http://www.alhdc.org.za.

Agamben, Giorgio. 1998. *Homo Sacer: Sovereign Power and Bare Life*. Stanford, CA: Stanford University Press.

Akrich, Madeleine. 1992. "The De-Scription of Technical Objects." In *Shaping Technology/Building Society: Studies in Sociotechnical Change*, ed. Wiebe E. Bijker and John Law, 20–24. Cambridge, MA: MIT Press.

Anderson, Warwick. 2003. "How's the Empire? An Essay Review." *Journal of the History of Medicine* 58 (4): 459–465.

Appadurai, Arjun. 2004. "The Capacity to Aspire: Culture and the Terms of Recognition." In *Culture and Public Action*, edited by Vijayendra Rao and Michael Walton, 59–84. Stanford, CA: Stanford University Press.

Appiah, Kwame Anthony. 2020. "The Case for Capitalizing the B in Black." *The Atlantic*, June 18, 2020.

Apple, Rima. 1987. *Mothers and Medicine: A Social History of Infant Feeding, 1890–1950*. Madison: University of Wisconsin Press.

Ardington, Cally, and Anne Case. "Health: Analysis of the NIDS Wave 1 Dataset, Discussion Paper no. 2." Cape Town: Southern African Labour and Development Research Unit. 2009.

Ashforth, Adam. 2005. *Witchcraft, Violence, and Democracy in South Africa*. Chicago: University of Chicago Press.

Attwell, David. 1992. *Doubling the Point: Essays and Interviews*. Cambridge, MA: Harvard University Press.

Bac, Martin, and Ingrid I. Glatthaar. 1990. "Protein-Energy Malnutrition Intervention Strategies." *South African Family Practice* 11: 284–291.

Baer, Hans A. 2012. "Engaged Anthropology in 2011: A View from the Antipodes in a Turbulent Era." *American Anthropologist* 114 (2): 217–226. https://doi.org/10.1111/j.1548-1433.2012.01420.x.

Baird, Barbara. 2008. "Child Politics, Feminist Analysis." *Australian Feminist Studies* 23: 291–305.

Barker, David J., and Clive Osmond. 1986. "Infant Mortality, Childhood Nutrition, and Ischaemic Heart Disease in England and Wales." *Lancet* 1 (8489): 1077–1081. https://doi.org/10.1016/S0140-6736(86)91340-1.

Basilico, Matthew, Jonathan Weigel, Anjali Motgi, Jacob Bor, and Salmaan Keshavjee. 2013. "Health for All? Competing Theories and Geopolitics." In *Reimagining Global Health: An Introduction*, edited by Paul Farmer, Jim Yong Kim, Arthur Kleinman, and Matthew Basilico, 7–10. Berkeley: University of California Press.

Bateson, Patrick. 2001. "Fetal Experience and Good Adult Design." *International Journal of Epidemiology* 30: 928–934.

Battersby, Jane. 2011. *The State of Urban Food Security in Cape Town*. Urban Food Security Series No. 11. Kingston and Cape Town: Queen's University and AFSUN. 2011.

Bauer, Susanne. 2013. "Modeling Population Health." *Medical Anthropology Quarterly* 27 (4): 510–530. https://doi.org/10.1111/maq.12054.

Baumann, Zygmunt. 1989. *Modernity and the Holocaust*. Cambridge: Polity Press.

Bayart, Jean-Francois. 1993. *The State in Africa: The Politics of the Belly*. London: Longman.

Beck, Ulrich. 1992. *Risk Society: Towards a New Modernity*. London: SAGE.

Beinart, William, and Saul Dubow, eds. 1995. *Segregation and Apartheid in Twentieth Century South Africa*. London: Routledge.

Ben-Shlomo, Yoav, Rachel Cooper, and Diana Kuh. 2016. "The Last Two Decades of Life Course Epidemiology, and Its Relevance for Research on Ageing." *International Journal of Epidemiology* 45 (4): 973–988. https://doi.org/10.1093/IJE/DYW096.

Benyshek, Daniel C. 2007. "The Developmental Origins of Obesity and Related Health Disorders—Prenatal and Perinatal Factors." *Collegium Antropologicum* 31 (1): 11–17. http://www.ncbi.nlm.nih.gov/pubmed/17598381.

Benyshek, Daniel C., John F. Martin, and Carol S. Johnston. 2001. "A Reconsideration of the Origins of the Type 2 Diabetes Epidemic among Native Americans and the Implications for Intervention Policy." *Medical Anthropology* 20 (1): 37–41. https://doi.org/10.1080/01459740.2001.9966186.

Berger, Shelley L., Tony Kouzarides, Ramin Shiekhattar, and Ali Shilatifard. 2009. "An Operational Definition of Epigenetics." *Genes and Development* 23: 781–783. https://doi.org/10.1101/gad.1787609.

Berlant, Lauren. 1998. "Intimacy: A Special Issue." *Critical Inquiry* 24 (2): 281–288.

———. 2007. "Slow Death (Sovereignty, Obesity, Lateral Agency)." *Critical Inquiry* 33 (4): 754–780. https://doi.org/10.1086/521568.

———. 2011. *Cruel Optimism*. Durham, NC: Duke University Press.

Bezuidenhout, Vincent. 2011. "Separate Amenities: Topographics of Recreational Spaces in South Africa." MA thesis, University of Cape Town.

Biehl, João G., and Adriana Petryna, eds. 2013. *When People Come First: Critical Studies in Global Health*. Princeton, NJ: Princeton University Press.

Black, Robert E., Cesar G. Victora, Susan P. Walker, Zulfiqar A. Bhutta, Parul Christian, Mercedes de Onis, Majid Ezzati, et al. 2013. "Maternal and Child Undernutrition and Overweight in Low-Income and Middle-Income Countries." *Lancet* 6736 (13): 427–451. https://doi.org/10.1016/S0140-6736(13)60937-X.

Bodenhorn, Barbara and Gabriele vom Bruck. 2006. "'Entangled in Histories': An Introduction to the Anthropology of Names and Naming." In *An Anthropology of Names and Naming*, edited by Gabriele vom Bruck and Barbara Bodenhorn, 1–30. Cambridge: Cambridge University Press.

Boese, Stefanie. 2017. "J. M. Coetzee's *Disgrace* and the Temporality of Injury." *Critique: Studies in Contemporary Fiction* 58 (3): 248–257. https://doi.org/10.1080/00111619.2016.1211985.

Bond, Patrick. 2007. "South Africa between Neoliberalism and Social Democracy? Respecting Balance While Sharpening Differences." *Politikon* 34 (2): 125–146. https://doi.org/10.1080/02589340701715182.

Bonduriansky, Russell. 2012. "Rethinking Heredity, Again." *Trends in Ecology & Evolution* 27 (6): 330–336.

Bourne, Lesley T., M. L. Langenhoven, Krisela Steyn, P. L. Jooste, J. A. Laubscher, and E. Van der Vyver. 1994. "Nutrient Intake in the Urban African Population of the Cape Peninsula, South Africa. The BRISK Study." *The Central African Journal of Medicine* 39: 23–47.

Bourne, Lesley T., Estelle V. Lambert, and Krisela Steyn. 2002. "Where Does the Black Population of South Africa Stand on the Nutrition Transition?" *Public Health Nutrition* 5 (1A): 157–162.

Breckenridge, Keith. 2014. *Biometric State: The Global Politics of Identification and Surveillance in South Africa, 1850 to the Present.* Cambridge: Cambridge University Press.

Brives, Charlotte. 2013. "Identifying Ontologies in a Clinical Trial." *Social Studies of Science* 43 (3): 397–416.

Brown, Hannah. 2016. "Managerial Relations in Kenyan Health Care: Empathy and the Limits of Governmentality." *Journal of the Royal Anthropological Institute* 22 (3): 591–609. https://doi.org/10.1111/1467-9655.12448.

Brunn, Stanley D., and Matthew W. Wilson. 2013. "Cape Town's Million Plus Black Township of Khayelitsha: Terrae Incognitae and the Geographies and Cartographies of Silence." *Habitat International* 39 (July): 284–294. https://doi.org/10.1016/j.habitatint.2012.10.017.

Bryce, Jennifer, Denise Coitinho, Ian Darnton-Hill, David Pelletier, and Per Pinstrup-Andersen. 2008. "Maternal and Child Undernutrition: Effective Action at National Level." *Lancet* 371 (9611): 510–526. https://doi.org/10.1016/S0140-6736(07)61694-8.

Burman, Erica. 1994. "Innocents Abroad: Western Fantasies of Childhood and the Iconography of Emergencies." *Disasters* 18 (3): 238–253. https://doi.org/10.1111/j.1467-7717.1994.tb00310.x.

Burman, Sandra, and Pamela Reynolds, eds. 1986. *Growing up in a Divided Society.* Johannesburg: Ravan Press.

Burns, Catherine E. 1995. "Reproductive Labors: The Politics of Women's Health in South Africa, 1900 to 1960." PhD diss., Northwestern University.

Burton, Rosie, Janet Giddy, and Kathryn Stinson. 2015. "Prevention of Mother-to-Child Transmission in South Africa: An Ever-Changing Landscape." *Obstetric Medicine* 8 (1): 5–12. https://doi.org/10.1177/1753495X15570994.

Buthelezi, Ernest P., Maria Terésa van der Merwe, Peter N. Lönnroth, I. Peter Gray, and Nigel J. Crowther. 2000. "Ethnic Differences in the Responsiveness of Adipocyte Lipolytic Activity to Insulin." *Obesity Research* 8 (2): 171–178.

Caduff, Carlo. 2014. "Pandemic Prophecy, or How to Have Faith in Reason." *Current Anthropology* 55 (3): 296–315. https://doi.org/10.1086/676124.

Caldwell, John C. 1976. "Toward a Restatement of Demographic Transition Theory." *Population and Development Review* 2 (3/4): 321–366. https://doi.org/10.2307/1971615.

Canguilhem, George. 1978. *On the normal and the pathological.* Boston: D Reidel.

———. 2008. *Knowledge of Life.* Translated by Stefanos Geroulanos and Daniela Ginsburg. Edited by Paola Marrati and Todd Meyers. New York: Fordham University Press.

Cape Town Tourism. 2015. "Khayelitsha Township Tour." Accessed February 1, 2016. http://www.capetown.travel/attractions/entry/Khayelitsha_Township_Tour_and_Craft_Market.

Carney, Megan A. 2015. "Eating and Feeding at the Margins of the State: Barriers to Health Care for Undocumented Migrant Women and the 'Clinical' Aspects of Food Assistance." *Medical Anthropology Quarterly* 29 (2): 196–215. https://doi.org/10.1111/maq.12151.

Carolina, Martínez S., and Leal F. Gustavo. 2003. "Epidemiological Transition: Model or Illusion? A Look at the Problem of Health in Mexico." *Social Science & Medicine* 57 (3): 539–550. https://doi.org/10.1016/S0277-9536(02)00379-9.

Carsten, Janet. 2003. *After Kinship.* Cambridge: Cambridge University Press.

Castañeda, Claudia. 2002. *Figurations: Child, Bodies, Worlds.* Durham, NC: Duke University Press.

Castro, Arachu, and Laure Marchand-Lucas. 2000. "Does Authoritative Knowledge in Infant Nutrition Lead to Successful Breastfeeding? A Critical Perspective." In *Global Health*

Policy, Local Realities: The Fallacy of the Level Playing Field, edited by Linda M. Whiteford and Lenore Manderson, 23–64. Boulder: Lynne Rienner Publishers.

Chakrabarty, Dipesh. 1992. "Postcoloniality and the Artifice of History: Who Speaks for "Indian" Pasts?" *Representations*, no. 37: 1–26. http://www.jstor.org/stable/2928652.

Chatterji, Roma, Sangeeta Chattoo, and Veena Das. 1998. "The Death of the Clinic? Normality and Pathology in Recrafting Aging Bodies." In *Vital Signs: Feminist Reconfigurations of the Bio/Logical Body*, edited by Margrit Shildrick and Janet Price, 171–196. Edinburgh: Edinburgh University Press. https://doi.org/10.1017/CBO9781107415324.004.

Chen, Lincoln C., Arthur Kleinman, and Norma C. Ware, eds. 1993. *Health and Social Change in International Perspective*. Boston: Harvard University Press.

City of Cape Town. 2014. "City's New Proposed Corporate Identity." Accessed August 14, 2014. https://www.capetown.gov.za/en/Pages/Cityproposednewcorporate identity.aspx.

Clarke, Adele E., Janet K. Shim, Laura Mamo, Jennifer Ruth Fosket, and Jennifer R. Fishman. 2003. "Biomedicalization: Technoscientific Transformations of Health, Illness, and U.S. Biomedicine." *American Sociological Review* 68 (2): 161–194.

Cleminshaw, Dot. 1985. "From Crossroads to Khayelitsha to . . . ?" *Reality* 18 (2): 11–14.

Coetzee, John M. 1999. *Disgrace*. London: Random House.

Cole, Josette. 1987. *Crossroads: The Politics of Reform and Repression, 1976–1986*. Johannesburg: Ravan Press.

Collins, Daryl, Jonathan Morduch, Stuart Rutherford, and Orlanda Ruthven. 2009. *Portfolios of the Poor: How the World's Poor Live on $2 a Day*. Princeton, NJ: Princeton University Press.

Comaroff, Jean, and John L. Comaroff. 2016. *The Truth about Crime: Sovereignty, Knowledge, Social Order*. Chicago: University of Chicago Press.

Connell, Raewyn. 2005. *Masculinities*. Berkeley: University of California Press.

Cooper, Melinda, and Catherine Waldby. 2014. *Clinical Labor: Tissue Donors and Research Subjects in the Global Bioeconomy*. Durham, NC: Duke University Press.

Cooper, P. J., Mark Tomlinson, Leslie Swartz, Mireille Landman, Chris Molteno, Alan Stein, Klim McPherson, and Lynne Murray. 2009. "Improving Quality of Mother-Infant Relationship and Infant Attachment in Socioeconomically Deprived Community in South Africa: Randomised Controlled Trial." *BMJ* 338 (b974): 1–8. https://doi.org/10.1136/bmj.b974.

Coovadia, Hoosen M. 1988. "What Is Progressive about PPHC?" In *Women's Health and Apartheid: The Health of Women and Children and the Future of Progressive Primary Health Care in Southern Africa: Proceedings of the Third Workshop of the Project on Poverty, Health, and the State in Southern Africa*, edited by Marcia Wright, Z. Stein, and J. Scandlyn, 293–298. New York: Columbia University.

Coovadia, Hoosen, Rachel Jewkes, Peter Barron, David Sanders, and Diane McIntyre. 2009. "The Health and Health System of South Africa: Historical Roots of Current Public Health Challenges." *Lancet* 374 (9692): 817–834. https://doi.org/10.1016/S0140-6736(09)60951-X.

Copenhagen Consensus Center. 2008. "Copenhagen Consensus 2008—Results." Copenhagen: Copenhagen Consensus Center. https://www.copenhagenconsensus.com/sites /default/files/cc08_results_final_0.pdf.

Cousins, Thomas. 2015. "HIV and the Remaking of Hunger and Nutrition in South Africa: Biopolitical Specification after Apartheid." *BioSocieties* 10 (2): 143–161. https://doi.org/10 .1057/biosoc.2015.8.

———. 2016. "Anti-Retroviral Therapy and Nutrition in Southern Africa: Citizenship and the Grammar of Hunger." *Medical Anthropology* 35 (5): 433–446. https://doi.org/10.1080 /01459740.2016.1141409.

———. 2023. *The Work of Repair: Capacity after Colonialism in the Timber Plantations of South Africa*. New York: Fordham University Press.

Cousins, Thomas, and Lindsey Reynolds. 2014. "Blood Relations: HIV Surveillance and Fieldworker Intimacy in KwaZulu-Natal, South Africa." In *Medical Anthropology in Global Africa*, edited by Kathryn Rhine, John M. Janzen, Glenn Adams, and Heather Aldersey, 79–88. Kansas: University of Kansas.

Coutsoudis, Anna, Kubendran Pillay, Elizabeth Spooner, Louise Kuhn, Hoosen M. Coovadia, and the South African Vitamin A Study Group. 1999. "Influence of Infant-Feeding Patterns on Early Mother-to-Child Transmission of HIV-1 in Durban, South Africa: A Prospective Cohort Study." *Lancet* 354: 471–476.

Crane, Johanna Tayloe. 2013. *Scrambling for Africa: AIDS, Expertise, and the Rise of American Global Health Science.* Ithaca, NY: Cornell University Press.

Darwin, Charles. 1859. *On the Origin of Species by Means of Natural Selection, or the Preservation of Favoured Races in the Struggle for Life.* London: Cassell and Company.

Das, Veena. 1995. *Critical Events: An Anthropological Perspective on Contemporary India.* Delhi: Oxford University Press.

———. 2007. *Life and Words: Violence and the Descent into the Ordinary.* Berkeley: University of California Press.

———. 2008. "Violence, Gender, and Subjectivity." *Annual Review of Anthropology* 37 (1): 283–99. https://doi.org/10.1146/annurev.anthro.36.081406.094430.

———. 2015. "Naming beyond Pointing: Singularity, Relatedness and the Foreshadowing of Death." *South Asia Multidisciplinary Academic Journal*, 12: 1–18. https://doi.org/10.4000/samaj.4005.

———. 2016. "The Boundaries of the 'We': Cruelty, Responsibility and Forms of Life." *Critical Horizons*, 17 (2): 168–185.

Das, Veena, and Ranendra K. Das. 2006. "Pharmaceuticals in Urban Ecologies: The Register of the Local." In *Global Pharmaceuticals: Ethics, Markets, Practices*, edited by Adriana Petryna, Andrew Lakoff, and Arthur Kleinman, 171–205. Durham, NC: Duke University Press.

Davin, Anna. 1978. "Imperialism and Motherhood." *History Workshop* 5: 9–65.

Dawber, Thomas R., and William B. Kannel. 1958. "An Epidemiologic Study of Heart Disease: The Framingham Study." *Nutrition Reviews* 16 (1): 1–4.

Deane, Kevin, and Sara Stevano. 2016. "Towards a Political Economy of the Use of Research Assistants: Reflections from Fieldwork in Tanzania and Mozambique." *Qualitative Research* 16 (2): 213–228.

DeBord, D. Gayle, Tania Carreón, Thomas J. Lentz, Paul J. Middendorf, Mark D. Hoover, and Paul A. Schulte. 2016. "Use of the 'Exposome' in the Practice of Epidemiology: A Primer on Omic Technologies." *American Journal of Epidemiology* 184 (4): 302–314. https://doi.org/10.1093/aje/kwv325.

De Lille, Patricia. 2014. "Cape Town's New Logo and Slogan Explained." Politicsweb. Accessed October 10, 2014. https://www.politicsweb.co.za/politics/cape-towns-new-logo-and-slogan-explained--patricia.

Delisle, Helen. 2002. *Programming of Chronic Disease by Impaired Fetal Nutrition: Evidence and Implications for Policy and Intervention Strategies.* Geneva: World Health Organisation.

Den Besten, Leo, Martin Bac, Ingrid I. Glatthaar, and Alexander R. Walker. 1995. "Changes in the Anthropometric Status of Rural African Under-Fives during a Decade of Primary Health Care." *The Journal of Tropical Medicine and Hygiene* 98 (6): 361–366. https://pubmed.ncbi.nlm.nih.gov/8544216/.

Department of Health, Republic of South Africa. 1998. *Integrated Nutrition Programme for South Africa. Summary of Broad Guidelines for Implementation.* Pretoria: Department of Health.

———.2013a. *Roadmap for Nutrition in South Africa 2013-2017.* Pretoria: Department of Health.

————. 2013b. *South African Infant and Young Child Feeding Policy 2013*. Pretoria: Department of Health.

————. 2015. *Guidelines for Maternity Care in South Africa. A Manual for Clinics, Community Health Centres and District Hospitals*. 4th ed. Pretoria: Department of Health.

Dewar, David, and Vanessa Watson. 1984. *The Concept of Khayelitsha: A Planning Perspective*. Cape Town: Urban Problems Research Unit, University of Cape Town.

Dewing, Sarah, Mark Tomlinson, Ingrid M. le Roux, Mickey Chopra, and Alexander C. Tsai. 2013. "Food Insecurity and Its Association with Co-Occurring Postnatal Depression, Hazardous Drinking, and Suicidality among Women in Peri-Urban South Africa." *Journal of Affective Disorders* 150 (2): 460–465. https://doi.org/10.1016/j.jad.2013.04.040.

Dickinson, Maggie. 2019. *Feeding the Crisis: Care and Abandonment in America's Food Safety Net*. Oakland: California University Press.

Dixon, Justin. 2012. "Protocol and Beyond: Practices of Care during a Tuberculosis Vaccine Clinical Trial in South Africa." *Anthropology Southern Africa* 35 (1–2): 40–48.

Dlamini, Jacob. 2009. *Native Nostalgia*. Auckland Park: Jacana.

Dolan, Catherine. 2012. "The New Face of Development: The 'Bottom of the Pyramid' Entrepreneurs." *Anthropology Today* 28 (4): 3–7. https://rai.onlinelibrary.wiley.com/doi/10.1111/j.1467-8322.2012.00883.x.

Donzelot, Jacques. 1979. *The Policing of Families*. New York: Pantheon.

Dörner, Günter. 1973. "Die mögliche bedeutung der prä- und/oder perinatalen ernährung für die pathogenese der obesitas." *Acta biologica et medica Germanica*, 30: 19–22.

Dörner, Günter, Elke Rodekamp, and Andreas Plagemann. 2008. "Maternal Deprivation and Overnutrition in Early Postnatal Life and Their Primary Prevention: Historical Reminiscence of an 'Ecological' Experiment in Germany." *Human Ontogenetics* 2: 51–59.

Douglas, Mary. 1992. *Risk and Blame: Essays in Cultural Theory*. New York: Routledge.

Du Toit, Andries, and David Neves. 2007. "In Search of South Africa's Second Economy: Chronic Poverty, Economic Marginalisation and Adverse Incorporation in Mt. Frere and Khayelitsha." Chronic Poverty Research Centre Working Paper No. 102, November 2007. http://dx.doi.org/10.2139/ssrn.1629206.

————. 2009. "Trading on a Grant: Integrating Formal and Informal Social Protection in Post-Apartheid Migrant Networks." Brooks World Poverty Institute Working Paper 75, January.

Du Toit, Andries, Andrew Skuse, and Thomas Cousins. 2007. "The Political Economy of Social Capital: Chronic Poverty, Remoteness and Gender in the Rural Eastern Cape." *Social Identities* 13 (4): 521–540. https://doi.org/10.1080/13504630701459180.

Dubois, Michel, and Catherine Guaspare. 2020. "From Cellular Memory to the Memory of Trauma: Social Epigenetics and Its Public Circulation." *Social Science Information* 59 (1): 144–183. https://doi.org/10.1177/0539018419897600.

Dubow, Saul. 1995. *Scientific Racism in Modern South Africa*. Cambridge: Cambridge University Press.

————. 2014. *Apartheid, 1948–1994*. Oxford: Oxford University Press.

————. 2017. "New Approaches to High Apartheid and Anti-Apartheid." *South African Historical Journal* 69 (2): 304–329. https://doi.org/10.1080/02582473.2017.1330896.

Duden, Barbara. 1993. *Disembodying Women: Perspectives on Pregnancy and the Unborn*. Cambridge, MA: Harvard University Press.

Durkheim, Emile. (1895) 1982. *The Rules of Sociological Method*. New York: Free Press.

Dwork, Deborah. 1987. *War Is Good for Babies and Other Young Children: A History of the Infant and Child Welfare Movement in England, 1899–1918*. London: Tavistock Publications.

Dworkin, Shari L., Abigail M. Hatcher, Chris Colvin, and Dean Peacock. 2012. "Impact of a Gender-Transformative HIV and Antiviolence Program on Gender Ideologies and Masculinities in Two Rural, South African Communities." *Men and Masculinities* 16 (2): 181–202. https://doi.org/10.1177/1097184X12469878.

Erasmus, Zimitri. 2008. "Race." In *New South African Keywords,* edited by Nick Shepherd and Steven Robins, 169–181. Johannesburg: Jacana.

Esposito, Roberto. 2008. *Bios: Biopolitics and Philosophy.* Minneapolis: Minnesota University Press.

Fassin, Didier. 2007. *When Bodies Remember: Experiences and Politics of AIDS in South Africa.* Berkeley: University of California Press.

———. 2012a. "That Obscure Object of Global Health." In *Medical Anthropology at the Intersections: Histories, Activisms, Futures,* edited by Marcia Inhorn and Emily A. Wentzell, 95–115. Durham, NC: Duke University Press.

———. 2012b. *Humanitarian Reason: A Moral History of the Present.* Berkeley: University of California Press.

———. 2013. "Children as Victims—The Moral Economy of Childhood in the Times of AIDS." In *When People Come First: Critical Studies in Global Health,* ed. João Guilherme Biehl and Adriana Petryna. 109–129. Princeton, NJ: Princeton University Press.

———. 2015. "Adventures of African Nevirapine: The Political Biography of a Magic Bullet." In *Para-States and Medical Science: Making African Global Health,* ed. Paul Wenzel Geissler, 33–54. Durham, NC: Duke University Press.

Fassin, Didier, Frédéric Le Marcis, and Todd Lethata. 2008. "Life & Times of Magda A." *Current Anthropology* 49 (2): 225–246. https://doi.org/10.1086/526096.

Feldman, Allen. 1995. "Ethnographic States of Emergency." In *Fieldwork under Fire: Contemporary Studies of Violence and Survival,* ed. Carolyn Nordstrom and Antonius C. G. M. Robben, 223–252. Berkeley: University of California Press.

Ferguson, James. 1999. *Expectations of Modernity: Myths and Meanings of Urban Life on the Zambian Copperbelt.* Berkeley: University of California Press.

———. 2015. *Give a Man a Fish: Reflections on the New Politics of Distribution.* Durham, NC: Duke University Press.

Fink, Günther, Evan Peet, Goodarz Danaei, Kathryn Andrews, Dana Charles McCoy, Christopher R. Sudfeld, Mary C. Smith Fawzi, et al. 2016. "Schooling and Wage Income Losses Due to Early-Childhood Growth Faltering in Developing Countries: National, Regional, and Global Estimates." *American Journal of Clinical Nutrition* 104: 104–112.

Fitz-James, Maximilian H., and Giacomo Cavalli. 2022. "Molecular Mechanisms of Transgenerational Epigenetic Inheritance." *Nature Reviews Genetics* 23 (6): 32–41.

Fleming, Paul J., Joseph G. L. Lee, and Shari L. Dworkin. 2014. "'Real Men Don't': Constructions of Masculinity and Inadvertent Harm in Public Health Interventions." *American Journal of Public Health* 104 (6): 1029–1035. https://doi.org/10.2105/AJPH.2013.301820.

Forsdahl, Anders. 1977. "Are Poor Living Conditions in Childhood and Adolescence an Important Risk Factor for Arteriosclerotic Heart Disease?" *British Journal of Preventive & Social Medicine* 31 (2): 91–95.

Foucault, Michel. 1970. *The Order of Things: an Archaeology of the Human Sciences.* London: Tavistock Publications.

———.1972. *The Archaeology of Knowledge and The Discourse on Language.* New York: Pantheon.

———. 1976. *The Birth of the Clinic: An Archeology of Medical Perception.* London: Tavistock Publications.

———. 1978. *The History of Sexuality*. Vol. 1, *The Will to Knowledge*. London: Penguin.

———. 1984. "What Is Enlightenment?" In *The Foucault Reader*, ed. Paul Rabinow, 32–50. New York: Pantheon.

———. 2003. *"Society Must Be Defended": Lectures at the College de France, 1975–76*. New York: Picador.

———. 2008. *The Birth of Biopolitics: Lectures at the College de France, 1978–1979*. New York: Palgrave Macmillan.

Fox, Graham R. 2012. "Race, Power and Polemic: Whiteness in the Anthropology of Africa." *Totem: The University of Ontario Journal of Anthropology* 20 (1): 10.

Frankenberg, Ruth. 1993. *White Women, Race Matters: The Social Construction of Whiteness*. Minneapolis: University of Minnesota Press.

Franklin, Sarah, and Faye Ginsburg. 2019. "Reproductive Politics in the Age of Trump and Brexit." *Cultural Anthropology* 34 (1): 3–9.

Freinkel, Norbert. 1980. "Of Pregnancy and Progeny." *Diabetes* 29 (12): 1023–1035.

Frenk, Julio, Jose L. Bobadilla, Jaime Sepulveda, and Malaquias Lopez. 1989. "Health Transition in Middle-Income Countries: New Challenges for Health Care." *Health and Policy Planning* 4 (1): 29–39.

Freund, Bill. 2011. "South Africa: The Union Years, 1910–1948—Political and Economic Foundations." In *The Cambridge History of South Africa*, vol. 2, *1885–1994*, edited by Robert Ross, Anne Kelk Mager, and Bill Nasson, 21–53. Cambridge: Cambridge University Press.

Gaitskell, Debbie. 1992. ""Getting Close to the Hearts of Mothers": Medical Missionaries among African Women and Children in Johannesburg between the Wars." In *Women and Children First: International Maternal and Infant Welfare, 1870–1945*, by Valerie Fildes, Lara Marks, and Hilary Marland, 33–72. London: Routledge.

Galton, Francis. 1869. *Hereditary Genius: An Inquiry into Its Laws and Consequences*. London: Macmillan.

Gálvez, Alyshia. 2018. *Eating NAFTA: Trade, Food Policies, and the Destruction of Mexico*. Oakland: University of California Press.

Geissler, Paul Wenzel. 2015. "Introduction: A Life Science in Its African Para-State." In *Para-States and Medical Science: Making African Global Health*, edited by Paul Wenzel Geissler, 1–44. Durham, NC: Duke University Press.

———. 2013a. "Public Secrets in Public Health: Knowing Not to Know While Making Scientific Knowledge." *American Ethnologist* 40 (1): 13–34. https://doi.org/10.1111/amet.12002.

———. 2013b. "The Archipelago of Public Health: Comments on the Landscape of Medical Research in Twenty-First Century Africa." In *Making and Unmaking Public Health in Africa: Ethnographic and Historical Perspectives*, edited by Ruth J. Prince and Rebecca Marsland, 23–55. Athens: Ohio University Press.

Geissler, Paul Wenzel, Ann Kelly, Babatunde Imoukhuede, and Robert Pool. 2008. "'He is now like a brother, I can even give him some blood'—Relational Ethics and Material Exchanges in a Malaria Vaccine "Trial Community" in The Gambia." *Social Science and Medicine* 67: 696–707.

Geissler, Paul Wenzel, and Guillaume Lachenal. 2016. "Brief Instructions for Archaeologists of African Futures." In *Traces of the Future: An Archaeology of Medical Science in Twenty-First Century Africa*, edited by Paul Wenzel Geissler, Guillaume Lachenal, John Manton, and Noemi Tousignant, 15–29. Chicago: University of Chicago Press.

Gibbs, Andrew, Cathy Vaughan, and Peter Aggleton. 2015. "Beyond 'Working with Men and Boys': (Re)Defining, Challenging and Transforming Masculinities in Sexuality and Health Programs and Policy." *Culture, Health & Sexuality* 17 (suppl. 2): 85–95. https://doi.org/10.1080/13691058.2015.1092260.

Gillespie, Kelly. 2014. "Murder and the Whole City." *Anthropology Southern Africa* 37 (3–4): 203–212.

Gillespie, Kelly, and Bernard Dubbeld. 2007. "The Possibility of a Critical Anthropology after Apartheid: Relevance, Intervention, Politics." *Anthropology Southern Africa* 30 (3–4): 129–134.

Gluckman, Peter D., and Mark A. Hanson. 2006. *Developmental Origins of Health and Disease.* Cambridge: Cambridge University Press.

Gluckman, Peter D., Mark A. Hanson, and Alan S. Beedle. 2007. "Non-Genomic Transgenerational Inheritance of Disease Risk." *Bioessays* 29: 145–154.

Gluckman, Peter D., Mark A. Hanson, and Tatjana Buklijas. 2010. "A Conceptual Framework for the Developmental Origins of Health and Disease." *Journal of Developmental Origins of Health and Disease* 1 (01): 6–18. https://doi.org/10.1017/S2040174409990171.

Gobodo-Madikizela, Pumla. 2016. "What Does It Mean to Be Human in the Aftermath of Mass Trauma and Violence? Toward the Horizon of an Ethics of Care." *Journal of the Society of Christian Ethics* 36 (2): 43–61. https://doi.org/10.1353/sce.2016.0030.

Godfrey, Keith M., Peter D. Gluckman, and Mark A. Hanson. 2010. "Developmental Origins of Metabolic Disease: Life Course and Intergenerational Perspectives." *Trends in Endocrinology and Metabolism* 21 (4): 199–205. https://doi.org/10.1016/j.tem.2009.12.008.

Godfrey, Keith M., Karen A. Lillycrop, Graham C. Burdge, Peter D. Gluckman, and Mark A. Hanson. 2007. "Epigenetic Mechanisms and the Mismatch Concept of the Developmental Origins of Health and Disease." *Pediatric Research* 61: 5–10. https://doi.org/10.1203/pdr.0b013e318045bedb.

Goldin, Ian. 1984. *The Poverty of Coloured Labour Preference: Economics and Ideology in the Western Cape.* Cape Town: Southern Africa Labour and Development Research Unit.

Good, Byron. 1994. *Medicine, Rationality and Experience.* Cambridge: Cambridge University Press.

Goodfellow, Aaron. 2014. "Pedagogies of the Clinic: Learning to Live (Again and Again)." In *Wording the World: Veena Das and Scenes of Instruction*, edited by Roma Chatterji, 3–4. New York: Fordham University Press.

Goodman, Alan H. 2013. "Bringing Culture into Human Biology and Biology Back into Anthropology." *American Anthropologist* 115 (3): 359–373. https://doi.org/10.1111/aman.12022.

Gottschang, Suzanne. 2000. "Reforming Routines: A Baby-Friendly Hospital in Urban China." In *Global Health Policy, Local Realities: The Fallacy of the Level Playing Field*, edited by Linda M. Whiteford and Lenore Manderson, 26–90. Boulder, CO: Lynne Rienner Publishers.

Gqola, Pulma Dineo. 2021. *Female Fear Factory.* Johannesburg: Melinda Ferguson.

Graham, Lucy Valerie. 2012. *State of Peril: Race and Rape in South African Literature.* Oxford: Oxford University Press.

Groenewald, Pamela, William Msemburi, Erna Morden, Nesbert Zinyakatira, Ian Neethling, Johann Daniels, Juliet Evans, et al. 2014. *Western Cape Mortality Profile 2011.* Cape Town: South African Medical Research Council.

Grossniklaus, Ueli, William G. Kelly, Bill Kelly, Anne C. Ferguson-Smith, Marcus Pembrey, and Susan Lindquist. 2013. "Transgenerational Epigenetic Inheritance: How Important Is It?" *Nature Reviews: Genetics* 14 (3): 228–235. https://doi.org/10.1038/nrg3435.

Guma, Mthobeli. 2001. "The Cultural Meaning of Names among Basotho of Southern Africa: A Historical and Linguistic Analysis." *Nordic Journal of African Studies* 10 (3): 265–279.

Gupta, Akhil. 2012. *Red Tape: Bureaucracy, Structural Violence, and Poverty in India.* Durham, NC: Duke University Press.

Guyer, Jane I. 1981. "Household and Community in African Studies." *African Studies Review* 24 (2): 87–137.

———. 2007. "Prophecy and the Near Future: Thoughts on Macroeconomic, Evangelical, and Punctuated Time." *American Ethnologist* 34 (3): 409–421. https://doi.org/10.1525/ae.2007.34.3.409.

Ha, Thu-Huong. 2018. "Bilingual Authors Are Challenging the Practice of Italicizing Non-English Words." Quartz. Accessed January 3, 2023. https://qz.com/quartzy/1310228/bilingual-authors-are-challenging-the-practice-of-italicizing-non-english-words.

Haddad, Lawrence. 2012. "The African Nutrition Congress: Declare the End of the 22nd Century Mindset." Development Horizons, October 3. Accessed May 10, 2016. http://www.developmenthorizons.com/2012/10/the-african-nutrition-congress-declare.html.

Hage, Ghassan. 2003. *Against Paranoid Nationalism*. Melbourne: Pluto Press.

———. 2009. "Waiting out the Crisis: On Stuckedness and Governmentality." In *Waiting*, ed. Ghassan Hage, 97–106. Melbourne: Melbourne University Press.

Hales, C. Nicholas, and David J. P. Barker. 1992. "Type 2 (Non-Insulin-Dependent) Diabetes Mellitus: The Thrifty Phenotype Hypothesis." *Diabetologia* 35: 595–601.

Hall, Katharine, and Dorrit Posel. 2019. "Fragmenting the Family? The Complexity of Household Migration Strategies in Post-Apartheid South Africa." *IZA Journal of Development and Migration* 10 (4). https://doi.org/10.2478/izajodm-2019-0004.

Han, Clara. 2012. *Life in Debt: Times of Care and Violence in Neoliberal Chile*. Berkeley: University of California Press.

Hanna, Bridget, and Arthur Kleinman. 2013. "Unpacking Global Health: Theory and Critique." In *Reimagining Global Health: An Introduction*, ed. Paul Farmer, Arthur Kleinman, J. Kim, and M. Basilico, 15–32. Berkeley: University of California Press.

Hansen, Tine T., Marietjie Herselman, Lisanne du Plessis, Luzette Daniels, Tirsa Bezuidenhout, Cora van Niekerk, Laura Truter, and Per O. Iversen. 2015. "Evaluation of Selected Aspects of the Nutrition Therapeutic Program Offered to HIV-Positive Women of Child-Bearing Age in Western Cape Province, South Africa." *Southern African Journal of HIV Medicine* 16 (1): 1–5. https://doi.org/10.4102/sajhivmed.v16i1.338.

Haraway, Donna. 1990. *Primate Visions: Gender, Race, and Nature in the World of Modern Science*. New York: Routledge.

———. 1997. *Modest_witness@second_ millennium. Femaleman_ meets_oncomouse*. New York: Routledge.

Hastrup, Kirsten, Peter Elsass, Ralph Grillo, Per Mathiesen, and Robert Paine. 1990. "Anthropological Advocacy: A Contradiction in Terms." *Current Anthropology* 31 (3): 301–311.

Hatch, Michelle, and Dorrit Posel. 2018. "Who Cares for Children? A Quantitative Study of Childcare in South Africa." *Development Southern Africa* 35 (2): 267–282. https://doi.org/10.1080/0376835X.2018.1452716.

Heard, Edith, and Robert A. Martienssen. 2014. "Transgenerational Epigenetic Inheritance: Myths and Mechanisms." *Cell* 157 (1): 95–109. https://doi.org/10.1016/j.immuni.2010.12.017.

Hedlund, Maria. 2011. "Epigenetic Responsibility." *Medicine Studies* 3 (3): 171–183. https://doi.org/10.1007/s12376-011-0072-6.

Heijmans, Bastiaan T., Elmar W. Tobi, Aryeh D. Stein, Hein Putter, Gerard J. Blauw, Ezra S. Susser, P. Eline Slagboom, and L. H. Lumey. 2008. "Persistent Epigenetic Differences Associated with Prenatal Exposure to Famine in Humans." *Proceedings of the National Academy of Sciences of the United States of America* 105 (44): 17046–17049. https://doi.org/10.1073/pnas.0806560105.

Helman, Rebecca, and Kopano Ratele. 2016. "Everyday (In)Equality at Home: Complex Constructions of Gender in South African Families." *Global Health Action* 9 (1). https://doi.org/10.3402/gha.v9.31122.

Herrick, Clare. 2017. "When Places Come First: Suffering, Archetypal Space and the Problematic Production of Global Health." *Transactions of the Institute of British Geographers* 42 (4): 530–543. https://doi.org/10.1111/tran.12186.

Heslehurst, Nicola, Rute Vieira, Zainab Akhter, Hayley Bailey, Emma Slack, Lem Ngongalah, Augustina Pemu, and Judith Rankin. 2019. "The Association between Maternal Body Mass Index and Child Obesity: A Systematic Review and Meta-Analysis." *PLoS Medicine* 16 (6): e1002817. https://doi.org/10.1371/journal.pmed.1002817.

———. 2013. "Dereliction at the South African Department of Home Affairs: Time for the Anthropology of Bureaucracy." *Critique of Anthropology* 1: 1–11. https://doi.org/10.1177/0308275X14543395.

Holmes, Peter and Michael Meadows (eds). 2012. *Southern African Geomorphology: Recent Trends and New Directions*. Bloemfontein: Sun Media.

Hoosain, Shanaaz. 2013. "The Transmission of Intergenerational Trauma in Displaced Families." PhD diss., University of the Western Cape.

Hopper, Kim. 2013. "The Murky Middle Ground—When Ethnographers Engage Public Health." *Social Science & Medicine* 99 (December): 201–204. https://doi.org/10.1016/j.socscimed.2013.10.025.

Huchzermeyer, Marie. 2003. "Low Income Housing and Commodified Urban Segregation in South Africa." In *Ambiguous Restructurings of Post-Apartheid Cape Town: The Spatial Form of Socio-Political Change*, edited by C. Haferburg and J. Oßenbrugge, 11–36. London: LitVerlag.

Hunt, Nancy Rose. 1999. *A Colonial Lexicon: Of Birth Ritual, Medicalization, and Mobility in the Congo*. Durham, NC: Duke University Press.

———. 2016. *A Nervous State*. Durham, NC: Duke University Press.

Hunter, Mark. 2010. *Love in the Time of AIDS. Inequality, Gender, and Rights in South Africa*. Pietermaritzburg: University of KwaZulu-Natal Press.

———. 2015. "Schooling Choice in South Africa: The Limits of Qualifications and the Politics of Race, Class and Symbolic Power." *International Journal of Educational Development* 43: 41–50. https://doi.org/10.1016/j.ijedudev.2015.04.004.

Igumbor, Ehimario U., David Sanders, Thandi R. Puoane, Lungiswa Tsolekile, Cassandra Schwarz, Christopher Purdy, Rina Swart, et al. 2012. "'Big Food,' the Consumer Food Environment, Health, and the Policy Response in South Africa." *PLoS Medicine* 9 (7): e1001253. https://doi.org/10.1371/journal.pmed.1001253.

Ijumba, Petrida, Tanya Doherty, Debra Jackson, Mark Tomlinson, David Sanders, and Lars-Åke Persson. 2013. "Free Formula Milk in the Prevention of Mother-to-Child Transmission Program: Voices of a Peri-Urban Community in South Africa on Policy Change." *Health Policy and Planning* 28 (7): 761–768. https://doi.org/10.1093/heapol/czs114.

Ingold, Tim, and Gisli Palsson. 2013. *Biosocial Becomings: Integrating Social and Biological Anthropology*. Cambridge: Cambridge University Press.

IRIN. 2012. "Nutrition Getting the Attention It Deserves?" *The New Humanitarian*, October 31. Accessed January 20, 2017. https://www.thenewhumanitarian.org/news/2012/10/31/nutrition-getting-attention-it-deserves.

Jablonka, Eva, and Marion J. Lamb. 2002. "The Changing Concept of Epigenetics." *Annals of the New York Academy of Sciences* 981 (1): 82–96. https://doi.org/10.1111/j.1749-6632.2002.tb04913.x.

James, Deborah. 2014. *Money from Nothing: Indebtedness and Aspiration in South Africa.* Johannesburg: Wits University Press.

Jasienska, Grazyna. 2009. "Low Birth Weight of Contemporary African Americans: An Intergenerational Effect of Slavery?" *American Journal of Human Biology* 21: 16–24. https://doi.org/10.1002/ajhb.20824.

Jeliffe, Derrick B. 1972. "Commerciogenic Malnutrition?" *Nutrition Reviews* 30: 199–205.

Jensen, Steffen. 2008. *Gangs, Politics & Dignity in Cape Town.* Chicago: University of Chicago Press.

Jewkes, Rachel, and Robert Morrell. 2012. "Sexuality and the Limits of Agency among South African Teenage Women: Theorising Femininities and Their Connections to HIV Risk Practices." *Social Science & Medicine* 74 (11): 1729–1737. https://doi.org/10.1016/j.socscimed.2011.05.020.

Jobson, Ryan Cecil. 2020. "The Case for Letting Anthropology Burn: Sociocultural Anthropology in 2019." *American Anthropologist* 122 (2): 259–271. https://doi.org/10.1111/aman.13398.

Johnson-Hanks, Jennifer. 2005. "When the Future Decides." *Current Anthropology* 46 (3): 363–385. https://doi.org/10.1086/428799.

Joseph, K. S., and Michael S. Kramer. 1996. "Review of the Evidence on Fetal and Early Childhood Antecedents of Adult Chronic Disease." *Epidemiologic Reviews* 18 (2): 158–174.

Joubert Jané, Rosana Norman, Debbie Bradshaw, Julia H. Goedecke, Nelia P. Steyn, Thandi Puoane and the South African Comparative Risk Assessment Collaborating Group. 2007. "Estimating the Burden of Disease Attributed to Excess Weight in South Africa in 2000." *South African Medical Journal* 97(8, Pt 2): 683–690.

Joyce, Andrew R., and Bernhard Ø. Palsson. 2006. "The Model Organism as a System: Integrating "Omics" Data Sets." *Nature Reviews Molecular Cell Biology* 7 (3): 198–210. https://doi.org/10.1038/nrm1857.

Kaati, Gunnar, Bygren, Lars O., and Sörren Edvinsson. 2002. "Cardiovascular and Diabetes Mortality Determined by Nutrition during Parents' and Grandparents' Slow Growth Period." *European Journal of Human Genetics* 10 (11): 682–688. https://doi.org/10.1038/sj.ejhg.5200859.

Kalemba, Joshua. 2020. "'Being Called Sisters': Masculinities and Black Male Nurses in South Africa." *Gender, Work and Organization* 27 (4): 647–663. https://doi.org/10.1111/gwao.12423

Kalofonos, Ippolytos Andreas. 2010. "'All I eat is ARVs': The Paradox of AIDS Treatment Interventions in Central Mozambique." *Medical Anthropology Quarterly* 24 (3): 363–380. https://doi.org/10.1111/j.1548-1387.2010.01109.x.

Kalumba, Phumzile Simelane. 2017. *Jabulani Means Rejoice: A Dictionary of South African Names.* Cape Town: Modjaji.

Kannel, William B., Thomas F. Dawber, Abraham Kagan, Nicholas Revotskie, and James Stokes III. 1961. "Factors of Risk in Development of Coronary Heart Disease–Six Year Follow-Up Experience: The Framingham Study." *Annals of Internal Medicine* 55: 33–50.

Kautzky, Keegan, and Stephen M. Tollman. 2008. "A Perspective on Primary Health Care in South Africa." In *South African Health Review 2008*, edited by P. Barron and J. Roma-Reardon, 17–30. Durban: Health Systems Trust.

Keller, Evelyn Fox. 2000. *The Century of the Gene.* Cambridge, MA: Harvard University Press.

Kenney, Martha, and Ruth Müller. 2017. "Of Rats and Women: Narratives of Motherhood in Environmental Epigenetics." *BioSocieties* 12 (1): 23–46.

Kermack, William O., Anderson G. McKendrick, and Peter L. McKinlay. 1934. "Death-Rates in Great Britain and Sweden. Some General Regularities and Their Significance." *Lancet* 223 (5770): 698–703. https://doi.org/10.1016/S0140-6736(00)92530-3.

Khan, Themrise, Seye Abimbola, Catherine Kyobutungi, and Madhukar Pai. 2022. "How We Classify Countries and People—and Why It Matters." *BMJ Global Health* 7 (6): e009704. http://dx.doi.org/10.1136/bmjgh-2022-009704.

Khayelitsha Commission. 2014. *Towards a Safer Khayelitsha: The Report of the Commission of Enquiry into Allegations of Police Inefficiency and a Breakdown in Relations between SAPS and the Community in Khayelitsha.* Cape Town: Commission of Inquiry into Allegations of Police Inefficiency and a Breakdown in Relations between SAPS and the Community in Khayelitsha. https://www.westerncape.gov.za/files/khayelitsha_commission_report.pdf.

Kleinman, Arthur. 1995. *Writing at the margin: discourse between anthropology and medicine.* Berkeley: University of California Press.

Kowal, Emma, and Megan Warin. 2018. "Anthropology, Indigeneity, and the Epigenome." *American Anthropologist* 120 (4): 822–835.

Krieger, Nancy. 2011. *Epidemiology and the People's Health: Theory and Context.* Oxford: Oxford University Press.

Kruger, H. Salome, Thandi Puoane, Marjanne Senekal, and M. T. van der Merwe. 2005. "Obesity in South Africa: Challenges for Government and Health Professionals." *Public Health Nutrition* 8 (5): 491–500. https://doi.org/10.1079/phn2005785.

Kruger, H. Salome, Christine S. Venter, and H. H. Vorster. 2001. "Obesity in African Women in the North West Province, South Africa Is Associated with an Increased Risk of Non-Communicable Diseases: The THUSA Study." *British Journal of Nutrition* 86 (6): 733–740.

Kruger, Lou-Marie. 2020. *Of Motherhood and Melancholia: Notebook of a Psycho-Ethnographer.* Pietermaritzburg: University of KwaZulu-Natal Press.

Kuh, Diana, Yoav Ben-Shlomo, John B. Lynch, Johan Hallqvist, and Christopher Power. 2003. "Life Course Epidemiology." *Journal of Epidemiology and Community Health* 57: 778–783.

Kuh, Diana, and George Davey Smith. 1993. "When Is Mortality Risk Determined? Historical Insights into a Current Debate." *Social History of Medicine* 6 (1): 101–123.

Kuhn, Louise, Merrick F. Zwarenstein, Geoffrey C. Thomas, Derek Yach, Hoffie H. Conradie, L. Hoogendoorn, and Judy M. Katzenellenbogen. 1990. "Village Health Workers and GOBI-FFF: An Evaluation of a Rural Program." *South African Medical Journal* 77 (5): 471–475.

Kuzawa, Christopher W., and Elizabeth Sweet. 2009. "Epigenetics and the Embodiment of Race: Developmental Origins of US Racial Disparities in Cardiovascular Health." *American Journal of Human Biology* 21 (1): 2–15. https://doi.org/10.1002/ajhb.20822.

Labadarios, Demetre, Nelia P. Steyn, C. Mgijima, and N. Daldla. 2005. "Review of the South African Nutrition Policy 1994–2002 and Targets for 2007: Achievements and Challenges." *Nutrition* 21 (January): 100–108. https://doi.org/10.1016/j.nut.2004.09.014.

Lachenal, Guillaume. 2015. "Lessons in Medical Nihilism: Virus Hunters, Neoliberalism, and the AIDS Pandemic in Cameroon." In *Para-States and Medical Science: Making African Global Health,* edited by Paul Wenzel Geissler. Durham, NC: Duke University Press.

Lambek, Michael. 2015. "Living as If It Mattered." In *Four Lectures on Ethics: Anthropological Perspectives,* edited by Michael Lambek, Veena Das, Didier Fassin, and Webb Keane, 1–33. Chicago: Hau Books.

Lambert, Helen, and Christopher McKevitt. 2002. "Anthropology in Health Research: From Qualitative Methods to Multidisciplinarity." *British Medical Journal* 325: 210.

Lamoreaux, Janelle. 2016. "What If the Environment Is a Person? Lineages of Epigenetic Science in a Toxic China." *Cultural Anthropology* 31 (2): 188–214. https://doi.org/10.14506/ca31.2.03.

Landecker, Hannah. 2011. "Food as Exposure: Nutritional Epigenetics and the New Metabolism." *BioSocieties* 6 (2): 167–194. https://doi.org/10.1057/biosoc.2011.1.

———. 2016. "Antibiotic Resistance and the Biology of History." *Body & Society* 22 (4): 19–52. https://doi.org/10.1177/1357034X14561341.

Landecker, Hannah, and Aaron Panofsky. 2013. "From Social Structure to Gene Regulation and Back: A Critical Introduction to Environmental Epigenetics for Sociology." *Annual Review of Sociology* 39: 333–357. https://doi.org/10.1146/annurev-soc-071312-145707.

Latour, Bruno. 1988. *The Pasteurization of France*. Cambridge, Mass: Harvard University Press.

Ledger, Tracey. 2016. "Hunger Feeds High Levels of Violence." BusinessDay, November 30. Accessed December 7, 2016. https://www.businesslive.co.za/bd/opinion/2016-11-30-hunger-feeds-high-levels-of-violence/#:~:text=Research%20shows%20that%20poor%20nutrition,control%20mechanisms%2C%20writes%20Tracy%20Ledger&text=Domestic%20violence%20levels%20in%20SA,cause%20for%20considerable%20national%20debate.

Le Marcis, Frédéric. 2004. "The Suffering Body of the City." *Public Culture* 16 (3): 453–477. https://doi.org/10.1215/08992363-16-3-453.

Le Marcis, Frédéric, and Julien Girard. 2015. "Ethnography of Everyday Ethics in a South African Medical Ward." In *Real Governance and Practical Norms in Sub-Saharan Africa: The Game of the Rules*, edited by Tom de Herdt and Jean-Pierre Olivier de Sardon. New York: Routledge.

Le Roux, Ingrid M., and P. J. Le Roux. 1991. "Survey of the Health and Nutrition Status of a Squatter Community in Khayelitsha." *South African Medical Journal* 79 (8): 500–503.

Lee, Rebekah. 2009. *African Women and Apartheid: Migration and Settlement in Urban South Africa*. London: Tauris Academic Studies.

Legassick, Martin, and Robert Ross. 2010. "From Slave Economy to Settler Capitalism: The Cape Colony and Its Extensions." In *The Cambridge History of South Africa*, vol. 1, *From Early Times to 1885*, edited by Carolyn Hamilton, Bernard K. Mbenga, and Robert Ross, 253–318. Cambridge: Cambridge University Press.

Leshabari, Sebalda C., Astrid Blystad, and Karen M. Moland. 2007. "Difficult Choices: Infant Feeding Experiences of HIV-Positive Mothers in Northern Tanzania." *SAHARA Journal* 4: 544–555.

Levine, Susan, Alison Swartz, and Hanna-Andrea Rother. 2020. "The Whistling of Rats." In *Connected Lives: Families, Households, Health and Care in South Africa*, edited by Nolwazi Mkhwanazi and Lenore Manderson, 12–24. Cape Town: HSRC Press.

Levitt, Naomi S., Judith M. Katzenellenbogen, Deborah Bradshaw, Margaret N. Hoffman, and Francois Bonnici. 1993. "The Prevalence and Identification of Risk Factors for NIDDM in Urban Africans in Cape Town, South Africa." *Diabetes Care* 16: 601–607.

Levitt, Naomi S., and Estelle V. Lambert. 2002. "The Foetal Origins of the Metabolic Syndrome—A South African Perspective." *Cardiovascular Journal of South Africa* 13 (4): 179–180.

Livingston, Julie. 2012. *Improvising Medicine: An African Oncology Ward in an Emerging Cancer Epidemic*. Durham, NC: Duke University Press.

Lock, Margaret. 1993. *Encounters with Ageing: Mythologies of Menopause in Japan and North America*. Berkeley: University of California Press.

———. 2005. "Eclipse of the gene and return of divination." *Current Anthropology*, 46 (S): S47–70.

———. 2013. "The Epigenome and Nature/Nurture Reunification: A Challenge for Anthropology." *Medical Anthropology* 32 (4): 291–308. https://doi.org/10.1080/01459740.2012.746973.

Lock, Margaret, and Gisli Palsson. 2016. *Can Science Resolve the Nature/Nurture Debate?* Cambridge: Polity Press.

MacGregor, Hayley. 2003. "Maintaining a Fine Balance: Negotiating Mental Distress in Khayelitsha, South Africa." PhD diss., University of Cambridge.

Maher, Jane Maree, Suzanne Fraser, and Jan Wright. 2010. "Framing the Mother: Childhood Obesity, Maternal Responsibility and Care." *Journal of Gender Studies* 19 (3): 233–247. https://doi.org/10.1080/09589231003696037.

Makhulu, Anna-Maria. 2010. "The Search for Economic Sovereignty." In *Hard Work, Hard Times: Global Volatility and African Subjectivities*, edited by Anna Maria Makhulu, Beth A. Buggenhagen, and Stephen Jackson, 2–7. Berkeley: University of California Press.

Malhotra, Rahul, Catherine Hoyo, Truls Østbye, Gail D. Hughes, D. Schwartz, Lungiswa Tsolekile, J. Zulu, and Thandi Puoane. 2008. "Determinants of Obesity in an Urban Township of South Africa." *South African Journal of Clinical Nutrition* 21 (4): 315–320.

Malkki, Liisa. 2015. *The Need to Help: The Domestic Arts of International Humanitarianism.* Durham, NC: Duke University Press.

Manderson, Lenore. 1982. "Bottle Feeding and Ideology in Colonial Malaya: The Production of Change." *International Journal of Health Services* 12 (4): 597–616.

Manderson, Lenore, and Fiona C. Ross. 2020. "Publics, Technologies and Interventions in Reproduction and Early Life in South Africa." *Humanities and Social Sciences Communications* 7 (1): 1–9. https://doi.org/10.1057/s41599-020-0531-3.

Manicom, Linzi. 1992. "Ruling Relations: Rethinking State and Gender in South African History." *Journal of African History* 33 (3): 441–465.

Mansfield, Becky. 2012. "Race and the New Epigenetic Biopolitics of Environmental Health." *BioSocieties* 7 (1): 352–372.

———. 2017. "Folded Futurity: Epigenetic Plasticity, Temporality, and New Thresholds of Fetal Life." *Science as Culture* 26 (3): 35–79.

Marks, Shula. 1994. *Divided Sisterhood: Race, Class and Gender in the South African Nursing Profession.* Johannesburg: Wits University Press.

Marks, Shula, and Neil Andersson. 1992. "Industrialisation, Rural Health and the 1944 National Health Services Commission in South Africa." In *The Social Basis of Health and Healing in Africa*, edited by Steven Feierman and John M. Janzen, 131–161. Berkeley: University of California Press.

Mascia-Lees, Frances E., and Patricia Sharpe. 2006. "Introduction to 'Cruelty, Suffering, Imagination: The Lessons of J. M. Coetzee.'" *American Anthropologist* 108 (1): 84–87.

Mathews, Eddie H., P. B. Taylor, M. Kleingeld, and M. F. Geyser. 2003. "Defining a New Condensation Boundary for Low-Cost Houses in South Africa." *Building and Environment* 38: 1475–84. https://doi.org/10.1016/S0360-1323(02)00035-5.

Maxwell, David. 2013. "The Durawall of Faith: Pentecostal Spirituality in Neo-Liberal Zimbabwe." *Journal of Religion in Africa* 35 (Fasc. 1): 4–32.

Mbembe, Achille. 2001. *On the Postcolony.* Berkeley: University of California Press.

Mbembe, Achille, and Janet Roitman. 1993. "Figures of the Subject in Times of Crisis." *Public Culture* 7: 323–352.

McKay, Ramah. 2018a. *Medicine in the Meantime: The Work of Care in Mozambique.* Durham, NC: Duke University Press.

———. 2018b. "Conditions of Life in the City: Medicine and Gendered Relations in Maputo, Mozambique." *Journal of the Royal Anthropological Institute* 24: 532–549.

McNaughton, Darlene. 2011. "From the Womb to the Tomb: Obesity and Maternal Responsibility." *Critical Public Health* 21 (2): 179–190. https://doi.org/10.1080/09581596.2010.523680.

Médecins Sans Frontières. 2011. *Scaling up Diagnosis and Treatment of Drug-Resistant Tuberculosis in Khayelitsha, South Africa.* Cape Town: Médecins Sans Frontières. https://msfaccess.org/sites/default/files/MSF_assets/TB/Docs/TB_report_ScalingUpDxTxKhaye_ENG_2011.pdf.

Mehlwana, Anthony. 1996. "The Dynamics of Cultural Continuities: Clanship in the Western Cape." MA diss., University of Cape Town.

Meinert, Lotte, and Lone Grøn. 2020. "'It Runs in the Family': Exploring Contagious Kinship Connections." *Ethnos* 85 (4): 581–594. https://doi.org/10.1080/00141844.2019.1640759.

Meloni, Maurizio. 2010. "Biopolitics for Philosophers." *Economy and Society* 39 (4): 551–566. https://doi.org/10.1080/03085147.2010.510684.

———. 2016. *Political Biology*. Basingstoke: Palgrave Macmillan.

Meloni, Maurizio, and Ruth Müller. 2018. "Transgenerational Epigenetic Inheritance and Social Responsibility: Perspectives from the Social Sciences." *Environmental Epigenetics* 4: 1–10.

Meloni, Maurizio, and Giuseppe Testa. 2014. "Scrutinizing the Epigenetics Revolution." *BioSocieties* 9 (4): 1–26. https://doi.org/10.1057/biosoc.2014.22.

Mengel, Ewald, and Michela Borzaga, eds. 2012. *Trauma, Memory, and Narrative in the Contemporary South African Novel: Essays*. Amsterdam: Rodopi.

Meyers, Todd. 2013. *The Clinic and Elsewhere: Addiction, Adolescents, and the Afterlife of Therapy*. Seattle: Washington University Press.

Mills, Elizabeth. 2016. "'You Have to Raise a Fist!' Seeing and Speaking to the State in South Africa." *IDS Bulletin* 47 (1): 69–82.

Mkhwanazi, Nolwazi. 2014. "'An African Way of Doing Things': Reproducing Gender and Generation." *Anthropology Southern Africa* 37 (1–2): 107–118. https://doi.org/10.1080/23323256.2014.969531.

———. 2016. "Medical Anthropology in Africa: The Trouble with a Single Story." *Medical Anthropology* 35 (2): 193–202. https://doi.org/10.1080/01459740.2015.1100612.

Mkhwanazi, Nolwazi, and Lenore Manderson, eds. 2020. *Connected Lives. Families, Households, Health and Care in Contemporary South Africa*. Cape Town: HSRC Press.

Mlungwana, Phumeza, and Dustin Kramer. 2019. *Fragments of Activism*. Cape Town: Blackman Rossouw Publishers.

Mofokeng, Lesley. 2012. *Bitch, Please! I'm Khanyi Mbau*. Cape Town: Tafelberg.

Mol, Annemarie. 2008. *The Logic of Care: Health and the Problem of Patient Choice*. New York: Routledge.

Moland, Karen Marie, and Astrid Blystad. 2009. "Counting on Mother's Love: The Global Politics of Prevention of Mother-to-Child Transmission of HIV in Eastern Africa." In *Anthropology and Public Health: Bridging Differences in Culture and Society*, edited by Robert A. Hahn and Marcia Inhorn, 44–79. Oxford: Oxford University Press.

Moore, Elena, and Jeremy Seekings. 2019. "Consequences of Social Protection on Intergenerational Relationships in South Africa: Introduction." *Critical Social Policy* 39 (4): 513–524. https://doi.org/10.1177/0261018319867582.

Morgan, Barak, Diane Sunar, C. Sue Carter, James F. Leckman, Douglas P. Fry, Eric B. Keverne, Iris-Tatjana Kolassa, et al. 2014. "Human Biological Development and Peace: Genes, Brains, Safety and Justice." In *Pathways to Peace: The Transformative Power of Children and Families*, edited by James F. Leckman, Catherine Panter-Brick, and Rima Salah, 95–128. Cambridge, MA: MIT Press.

Morgan, Barak, Robert Kumsta, Pasco Fearon, Dirk Moser, Sarah Skeen, Peter Cooper, Lynne Murray, et al. 2017. "Serotonin Transporter Gene (SLC6A4) Polymorphism and Susceptibility to a Home-visiting Maternal–Infant Attachment Intervention Delivered by Community Health Workers in South Africa: Reanalysis of a Randomized Controlled Trial." *PLOS Medicine* 14: e1002237.

Morreira, Shannon. 2012. "'Anthropological Futures?' Thoughts on Social Research and the Ethics of Engagement." *Anthropology Southern Africa* 35 (3–4): 100–104.

Morrell, Robert. 1998. "Of Boys and Men: Masculinity and Gender in Southern African Studies." *Journal of Southern African Studies* 24 (4): 605–630. https://doi.org/10.1080/03057079808708593.

Morrell, Robert, Rachel Jewkes, Graham Lindegger, and Vijay Hamlall. 2013. "Hegemonic Masculinity: Reviewing the Gendered Analysis of Men's Power in South Africa." *South African Review of Sociology* 44 (1): 3–21. https://doi.org/10.1080/21528586.2013.784445.

Mqombothi, Liduduma'lingani. 2014. "'Township' Is a Planet for Aliens." Africa Is a Country. Accessed April 22, 2014. http://africasacountry.com/2014/04/township-is-a-planet-for-aliens.

Mudimbé, Valentin-Yves. 1988. *The Invention of Africa: Gnosis, Philosophy, and the Order of Knowledge.* London: Currey.

Muchapondwa, Edwin. 2010. "A cost-effectiveness analysis of options for reducing pollution in Khayelitsha township, South Africa." *Journal for Transdisciplinary Research in Southern Africa* 6(2): 333–358.

Muller, Lauren. 2004. "The Geography of the Clinic: Spatial Strategies at a Western Cape Community Health Centre." *Anthropology Southern Africa* 27 (1–2): 54–63.

Müller-Wille, Staffan, and Hans Jörg Rheinberger. 2012. *A Cultural History of Heredity.* Chicago: University of Chicago Press.

Mulligan, Connie J. 2016. "Early Environments, Stress, and the Epigenetics of Human Health." *Annual Review of Anthropology* 45: 233–249. https://doi.org/10.1146/annurev-anthro-102215-095954.

Munn, Nancy D. 1992. "The Cultural Anthropology of Time: A Critical Essay." *Annual Review of Anthropology* 21 (1): 93–123. https://doi.org/10.1146/annurev.an.21.100192.000521.

Murphy, Elizabeth. 2000. "Risk, Responsibility, and Rhetoric in Infant Feeding." *Journal of Contemporary Ethnography* 29 (3): 291–325.

Murphy, Michelle. 2013. "Distributed Reproduction, Chemical Violence, and Latency." *Scholar and Feminist Online* 11 (3): 1–7.

———. 2017. *The Economization of Life.* Durham, NC: Duke University Press.

———. 2018. "Against Population, towards Alterlife." In *Making Kin Not Population*, edited by Adele E. Clarke and Donna Haraway. 101–124. Chicago: Prickly Paradigm Press.

Murray, Colin. 1987. "Displaced Urbanization: South Africa's Rural Slums." *African Affairs* 86 (344): 311–329.

Mvo, Zodumo, Judy Dick, and Krisela Steyn. 1999. "Perceptions of Overweight African Women about Acceptable Body Size of Women and Children." *Curationis* 22 (2): 27–31.

Myer, Landon, Rodney I. Ehrlich, and Ezra S. Susser. 2004. "Social Epidemiology in South Africa." *Epidemiologic Reviews* 26: 112–123.

Nattrass, Nicoli. 2008. "AIDS and the Scientific Governance of Medicine in Post-Apartheid South Africa." *African Affairs* 107 (427): 157–176.

Neely, Abigail H., and Alex M. Nading. 2017. "Global Health from the Outside: The Promise of Place-Based Research." *Health and Place* 45: 55–63.

Nestlé South Africa. 2013. "Magic on Wheels." Accessed August 16, 2013. http://www.nestle.co.za/csv/socioeconomicdevelopment/flagshipprogrammes/magiconwheels.

Nguyen, Vinh-Kim. 2005. "Antiretroviral Globalism, Biopolitics, and Therapeutic Citizenship." In *Global Assemblages: Technology, Politics, and Ethics as Anthropological Problems*, edited by Aihwa Ong and Stephen J. Collier. Oxford: Blackwell.

———. 2009. "Government-by-Exception: Enrolment and Experimentality in Mass HIV Treatment Programmes in Africa." *Social Theory & Health* 7 (3): 196–217. https://doi.org/http://dx.doi.org/10.1057/sth.2009.12.

———. 2010. *The Republic of Therapy: Triage and Sovereignty in West Africa's Time of AIDS.* Durham, NC: Duke University Press.

———. 2015. "Treating to Prevent HIV: Population Trials and Experimental Societies." In *Para-States and Medical Science: Making African Global Health*, edited by Paul Wenzel Geissler. Durham, NC: Duke University Press.

Ngwane, Zolani. 2003. "'Christmas Time' and the Struggles for the Household in the Country-side: Rethinking the Cultural Geography of Migrant Labour in South Africa." *Journal of Southern African Studies* 29 (3): 681–699. https://doi.org/10.1080/0305707032000094974.

Ngxiza, Sonwabile. 2012. "Sustainable Economic Development in Previously Deprived Local-ities: The Case of Khayelitsha in Cape Town." *Urban Forum* 23 (2): 181–195. https://doi .org/10.1007/s12132-011-9134-9.

Nichols, Carly E. 2019. "Geographic Contingency, Affective Facts, and the Politics of Global Nutrition Policy." *Geoforum* 105: 179–190.

Niehaus, Isak. 2013. *Witchcraft and a Life in the New South Africa*. Cambridge: Cambridge University Press.

Nieuwoudt, Sara, and Lenore Manderson. 2018. "Frontline Health Workers and Exclusive Breastfeeding Guidelines in an HIV Endemic South African Community: A Qualitative Exploration of Policy Translation." *International Breastfeeding Journal* 13: 20.

Nieuwoudt, Sara, Christian B. Ngandu, Lenore Manderson and Shane A. Norris. 2019. "Exclusive Breastfeeding Policy, Practice and Influences in South Africa, 1980 to 2018: A Mixed-Methods Systematic Review." *PLoS ONE* 14 (10): e0224029.

Niewöhner, Jörg. 2011. "Epigenetics: Embedded Bodies and the Molecularisation of Biography and Milieu." *Biosocieties* 6 (3): 279–298.

Niewöhner, Jörg, and Margaret Lock. 2018. "Situating Local Biologies: Anthropological Perspectives on Environment/Human Entanglements." *BioSocieties* 13: 681–697. https://doi .org/10.1057/s41292-017-0089-5.

Njuki, Jemimah, John R. Parkins, Amy Kaler and Sara Ahmed. 2016. "Introduction: Gender, Agriculture and Food Security: Where Are We?" In *Transforming Gender and Food Security in the Global South*, edited by Jemimah Njuki, John R. Parkins and Amy Kaler, 1–18. London: Routledge.

Nkomo, Nkululeko. 2015. "Bearing the Right to Healthcare, Autonomy and Hope." *Social Science & Medicine* 147: 163–169. https://doi.org/10.1016/j.socscimed.2015.11.003.

Nordstrom, Carolyn, and Antonius C. G. M. Robben. 1995. "Introduction: The Anthropology and Ethnography of Violence and Sociopolitical Conflict." In *Fieldwork under Fire*, edited by C. Nordstrom and A. Robben, 1–24. Berkeley: University of California Press.

Norris, Shane A., and Linda M. Richter. 2016. "The Importance of Developmental Origins of Health and Disease Research for Africa." *Journal of Developmental Origins of Health and Disease* 7 (2): 121–122.

Notkola, Veijo, Sven Punsar, Martti J. Karvonen, and Jaason Haapakoski. 1985. "Socio-Economic Conditions in Childhood and Mortality and Morbidity Caused by Coronary Heart Disease in Adulthood in Rural Finland." *Social Science & Medicine* 21 (5): 517–523.

Nuttall, Sarah, and Achille Mbembe, eds. 2008. *Johannesburg: The Elusive Metropolis*. Durham, NC: Duke University Press.

Nyamnjoh, Francis B. 2012. "Blinded by Sight: Divining the Future of Anthropology in Africa." *Africa Spectrum* 47 (2–3): 63–92.

———. 2015. "Beyond an Evangelising Public Anthropology: Science, Theory and Commit-ment." *Journal of Contemporary African Studies* 33 (1): 48–63.

Odunitan-Wayas, Feyisayo A., Kufre J. Okop, Robert V. H. Dover, Olufunke A. Alaba, Lisa K. Micklesfield, Thandi Puoane, Naomi S. Levitt, et al. 2021. "Food Purchasing Behaviour of Shoppers from Different South African Socio-Economic Communities: Results from

Grocery Receipts, Intercept Surveys and in-Supermarkets Audits." *Public Health Nutrition* 24 (4): 665–676.

Oldfield, Sophie, and Saskia Greyling. 2015. "Waiting for the State: A Politics of Housing in South Africa." *Environment and Planning A* 47 (5): 1100–1112. https://doi.org/10.1177/0308518X15592309.

Oldfield, Sophie, Netsai Sarah Matshaka, Elaine Salo, and Ann Schlyter. 2019. "In Bodies and Homes: Gendering Citizenship in Southern African Cities." *Urbani Izziv* 30: 37–51. https://doi.org/10.5379/urbani-izziv-en-2019-30-supplement-003.

Omran, Abdel. 1971. "The Epidemiological Transition: A Theory of the Epidemiology of Population Change." *Milbank Memorial Fund Quarterly* 49 (1): 509–538. https://www.ncbi.nlm.nih.gov/pmc/articles/PMC2690264/.

Ong, Aihwa. 1995. "Comment on The Primacy of the Ethical: Propositions for a Militant Anthropology." *Current Anthropology* 36 (3): 428–430.

Osmani, Siddiq, and Amartya Sen. 2003. "The Hidden Penalties of Gender Inequality: Fetal Origins of Ill-Health." *Economics and Human Biology* 1: 105–121.

Osterweil, Michael. 2013. "Rethinking Public Anthropology through Epistemic Politics and Theoretical Practice." *Cultural Anthropology* 28 (4): 598–620. https://doi.org/10.1111/cuan.12029.

Paneth, Nigel. 1994. "The Impressionable Fetus?" *American Journal of Public Health* 84: 1372–1374.

Peletz, Michael G. 2001. "Ambivalence in Kinship since the 1940s." In *Relative Values: Reconfiguring Kinship Studies*, edited by Sarah Franklin and Susan McKinnon, 41–44. Durham, NC: Duke University Press.

Pembrey, Marcus E., Lars Olov Bygren, Gunnar Kaati, Sören Edvinsson, Kate Northstone, Michael Sjöström, Jean Golding, and The ALSPAC Study Team. 2006. "Sex-Specific, Male-Line Transgenerational Responses in Humans." *European Journal of Human Genetics* 14: 159–66. https://doi.org/10.1038/sj.ejhg.5201538.

Penkler, Michael. 2022. "Caring for Biosocial Complexity: Articulations of the Environment in Research on the Developmental Origins of Health and Disease." *Studies in History and Philosophy of Science* 93: 1–10.

Pentecost, Michelle. 2018a. "Field Notes in the Clinic: On Medicine, Anthropology and Pedagogy in South Africa." *BMJ Medical Humanities* 44 (4): E1–E2. https://doi.org/10.1136/medhum-2018-011473.

———. 2018b. "The First Thousand Days: Epigenetics in the Age of Global Health." In *The Palgrave Handbook of Biology and Society*, edited by Maurizio Meloni, John Cromby, Des Fitzgerald, and Stephanie Lloyd, 269–294. London: Palgrave Macmillan.

Pentecost, Michelle, and Thomas Cousins. 2017. "Strata of the Political: Epigenetic and Microbial Imaginaries in Post-Apartheid Cape Town." *Antipode* 49 (5): 1368–1384. https://doi.org/10.1111/anti.12315.

———. 2018. "The Temporary as the Future: Ready-to-Use Therapeutic Food and Nutraceuticals in South Africa." *Anthropology Today* 34 (4): 9–13. https://doi.org/10.1111/1467-8322.12447.

———. 2019. "'The Good Doctor': The Making and Unmaking of the Physician Self in Contemporary South Africa." *Journal of Medical Humanities*. https://doi.org/10.1007/s10912-019-09572-y.

Pentecost, Michelle, and Maurizio Meloni. 2020. "'It's Never Too Early': Preconception Care and Postgenomic Models of Life." *Frontiers in Sociology* 5: 1–21. https://doi.org/10.3389/fsoc.2020.00021.

Pentecost, Michelle, and Fiona C. Ross. 2019. "The First Thousand Days: Motherhood, Scientific Knowledge, and Local Histories." *Medical Anthropology* 38 (8): 747–761. https://doi.org/10.1080/01459740.2019.1590825.

Petryna, Adriana. 2009. *When Experiments Travel: Clinical Trials and the Global Search for Human Subjects*. Princeton, NJ: Princeton University Press.

Pfeiffer, James. 2002. "African Independent Churches in Mozambique: Healing the Afflictions of Inequality." *Medical Anthropology Quarterly* 16 (2): 176–199. https://doi.org/10.1525/maq.2002.16.2.176.

Pickersgill, Martyn. 2016. "Epistemic Modesty, Ostentatiousness and the Uncertainties of Epigenetics: On the Knowledge Machinery of (Social) Science." *The Sociological Review Monograph* 64 (1): 186–202. https://doi.org/10.1111/2059-7932.12020.

Pickersgill, Martyn, Jörg Niewöhner, Ruth Müller, Paul Martin, and Sarah Cunningham-Burley. 2013. "Mapping the New Molecular Landscape: Social Dimensions of Epigenetics." *New Genetics and Society* 32 (4): 429–447. https://doi.org/10.1080/14636778.2013.861739.

Pinnock, Don. 2016. *Gang Town*. Cape Town: Tafelberg.

Plaatje, Sol T. (1916) 1995. *Native Life in South Africa: Before and since the European War and the Boer Rebellion*. Randburg: Ravan Press.

Popkin, Barry M. 1993. "Nutritional Patterns and Transitions." *Population and Development Review* 19 (1): 138–157.

Popkin, Barry M., Linda S. Adair, and Shu Wen Ng. 2011. "Global Nutrition Transition and the Pandemic of Obesity in Developing Countries." *Nutrition Reviews* 70 (1): 3–21. https://doi.org/10.1111/j.1753-4887.2011.00456.x.

Posel, Deborah. 1991. *The Making of Apartheid, 1948–1961: Conflict and Compromise*. Oxford: Clarendon Press.

———. 2001. "What's in a Name? Racial Categorisations under Apartheid and Their Afterlife." *Transformation: Critical Perspectives on Southern Africa* 47: 50–74.

Povinelli, Elizabeth A. 2006. *The Empire of Love: Toward a Theory of Intimacy, Genealogy, and Carnality*. Durham, NC: Duke University Press.

———. 2011. *Economies of Abandonment: Social Belonging and Endurance in Late Liberalism*. Durham, NC: Duke University Press.

Prestholdt, Jeremy. 2015. "Locating the Indian Ocean: Notes on the Postcolonial Reconstitution of Space." *Journal of Eastern African Studies* 9 (3): 440–467.

Ptashne, Mark. 2007. "On the Use of the Word 'Epigenetic.'" *Current Biology* 17 (7): R233–R236. https://doi.org/10.1016/j.cub.2007.02.030.

Punyadeera, Chamindie, M. T. van der Merwe, Nigel Crowther, Marketa Toman, A. R. Immelman, Glen P. Schlaphoff, and I. P. Gray. 2001. "Weight-Related Differences in Glucose Metabolism and Free Fatty Acid Production in Two South African Population Groups." *International Journal of Obesity and Related Metabolic Disorders* 25: 1196–1205.

Puoane, Thandi R., Krisela Steyn, Debbie Bradshaw, Ria Laubscher, Jean Fourie, Vicki Lambert, and Nolwazi Mbananga. 2002. "Obesity in South Africa: The South African Demographic and Health Survey." *Obesity Research* 10 (10): 1038–1048.

Puoane, Thandi R., Lungiswa Tsolekile, Ehimario U. Igumbor, and Jean M. Fourie. 2012. "Experiences in Developing and Implementing Health Clubs to Reduce Hypertension Risk among Adults in a South African Population in Transition." *International Journal of Hypertension* 2012: Article ID 913960. https://doi.org/10.1155/2012/913960.

Rabinbach, Anson. 1990. *The Human Motor: Energy, Fatigue, and the Origins of Modernity*. Berkeley: University of California Press.

Rabinow, Paul, and Nikolas Rose. 2006. "Biopower Today." *BioSocieties* 1 (2): 195–217. https://doi.org/10.1017/S1745855206040014.

Radcliffe-Brown, Alfred R., and Daryll Forde. 1950. *African Systems of Kinship and Marriage*. Oxford: Oxford University Press.

Radin, Joanna, and Noel Cameron. 2012. "Studying Mandela's Children: Human Biology in Post-Apartheid South Africa." *Current Anthropology* 53 (S5): S256–S266. https://doi.org/10.1086/662573.

Rajan, Kaushik Sunder. 2012. "Introduction: The Capitalization of Life and the Liveliness of Capital." In *Lively Capital: Biotechnologies, Ethics, and Governance in Global Markets*, edited by Kaushik Sunder Rajan, 1–4. Durham, NC: Duke University Press.

Reddy, Sasiragha, and Anthony Mbewu. 2016. "The Implications of the Developmental Origins of Health and Disease on Public Health Policy and Health Promotion in South Africa." *Healthcare* 4 (4): 83.

Ramphele, Mamphela. 1993. *A Bed Called Home: Life in the Migrant Labour Hostels of Cape Town*. Edinburgh: Edinburgh University Press.

Ratele, Kopano. 2016. *Liberating Masculinities*. Cape Town: HSRC Press.

Redfield, Peter. 2012. "Bioexpectations: Life Technologies as Humanitarian Goods." *Public Culture* 24 (1): 157–84. https://doi.org/10.1215/08992363-1443592.

Reed, Amber R. 2016. "Nostalgia in the Post-Apartheid State." *Anthropology Southern Africa* 39 (2): 97–109. https://doi.org/10.1080/23323256.2016.1172492.

Reynolds, Pamela. 1989. *Childhood in Crossroads: Cognition and Society in South Africa*. Cape Town: David Philip.

———. 2000. "The Ground of All Making: State Violence, the Family, and Political Activists." In *Violence and Subjectivity*, edited by Veena Das, Arthur Kleinman, Mamphela Ramphele, and Pamela Reynolds, 141–170. Berkeley: University of California Press.

———. 2013. *War in Worcester: Youth and the Apartheid State*. New York: Fordham University Press.

Rheinberger, Hans-Jörg. 2013. "Heredity in the Twentieth Century: Some Epistemological Considerations." *Public Culture* 25 (3): 477–494.

Richards, Audrey I. 1939. *Land, Labour and Diet in Northern Rhodesia: An Economic Study of the Bemba Tribe*. Oxford: Oxford University Press.

Richards, Eric J. 2006. "Inherited Epigenetic Variation—Revisiting Soft Inheritance." *Nature Reviews: Genetics* 7 (May): 395–402.

Richardson, Sarah S. 2015. "Maternal Bodies in the Postgenomic Order: Gender and the Explanatory Landscape of Epigenetics." In *Postgenomics: Perspectives on Biology and the Genome*, edited by S. S. Richardson and H. Stevens, 210–231. Durham, NC: Duke University Press.

Richter, Linda. 2022. *Birth to Thirty*. Wandsbeck: Reach Publishers.

Richter, Linda M., Cesar G. Victora, Pedro C. Hallal, Linda S. Adair, Santosh K. Bhargava, Caroline H. D. Fall, Nanette Lee, et al. 2012. "Cohort Profile: The Consortium of Health-Orientated Research in Transitioning Societies." *International Journal of Epidemiology* 41 (3): 621–26. https://doi.org/10.1093/ije/dyq251.

Richter, Linda, Shane Norris, John Pettifor, Derek Yach, and Noel Cameron. 2007. "Cohort Profile: Mandela's Children: The 1990 Birth to Twenty Study in South Africa." *International Journal of Epidemiology* 36 (3): 504–511. https://doi.org/10.1093/ije/dym016.

Rifkin, Susan B., and Gill Walt. 1986. "Why Health Improves: Defining the Issues Concerning 'Comprehensive Primary Health Care' and 'Selective Primary Health Care.'" *Social Science and Medicine* 23 (6): 559–66. https://doi.org/10.1016/0277-9536(86)90149-8.

Riggs, Damien, and Elizabeth Peel. 2016. *Critical Kinship Studies*. London: Palgrave.

Roberts, Dorothy. 2016. "The Ethics of Biosocial Science." The Tanner Lectures on Human Values. Delivered at Harvard University, November 2–3.

Robins, Steven. 2004. "'Long Live Zackie, Long Live': AIDS Activism, Science and Citizenship after Apartheid." *Journal of Southern African Studies* 30 (3): 651–672. https://doi.org/10.1080/0305707042000254146.

———. 2006. "From 'Rights' to 'Rituals': AIDS Activism in South Africa." *American Anthropologist* 108 (2): 312–23. https://doi.org/doi:10.1525/aa.2006.108.2.312.

———. 2014. "The 2011 Toilet Wars in South Africa: Justice and Transition between the Exceptional and the Everyday after Apartheid." *Development and Change* 45 (3): 479–501. https://doi.org/10.1111/dech.12091.

Rose, Nikolas. 2007. *The Politics of Life Itself: Biomedicine, Power, and Subjectivity in the Twenty-First Century*. Princeton, NJ: Princeton University Press.

Roseboom, Tessa J., Jan H. van der Meulen, Anita C. J. Ravelli, Clive Osmond, David J. Barker, and Otto P. Bleker. 2001. "Effects of Prenatal Exposure to the Dutch Famine on Adult Disease in Later Life: An Overview." *Twin Research* 4 (5): 293–298. https://doi.org/10.1375/1369052012605.

Ross, Fiona C. 2010. *Raw Life, New Hope: Decency, Housing and Everyday Life in a Post-Apartheid Community*. Cape Town: UCT Press.

———. 2015. "Raw Life and Respectability." *Current Anthropology* 56 (S11): S97–S107. https://doi.org/10.1086/682078.

Rottenburg, Richard. 2009. "Social and Public Experiments and New Figurations of Science and Politics in Postcolonial Africa." *Postcolonial Studies* 12 (4): 423–440. https://doi.org/10.1080/13688790903350666.

Roy, Deboleena. 2018. *Molecular Feminisms: Biology, Becoming and Life in the Lab*. Seattle: University of Washington Press.

Rubin, Margot. 2011. "Perceptions of Corruption in the South African Housing Allocation and Delivery Programme: What It May Mean for Accessing the State." *Journal of Asian and African Studies* 46 (5): 479–490. https://doi.org/10.1177/0021909611403706.

Saethre, Eirik, and Jonathan Stadler. 2017. *Negotiating Pharmaceutical Uncertainty: Women's Agency in a South African HIV Prevention Trial*. Nashville: Vanderbilt University Press.

Saldaña-Tejeda, Abril, and Peter Wade. 2019. "Eugenics, Epigenetics, and Obesity Predisposition among Mexican Mestizos." *Medical Anthropology* 38 (8): 66–79.

Salo, Elaine R. 2003. "Negotiating Gender and Personhood in the New South Africa." *European Journal of Cultural Studies* 6 (3): 345–365.

———. 2018. *Respectable Mothers, Tough Men and Good Daughters: Producing Persons in Manenberg Township South Africa*. Bamenda: Langaa RPCIG.

Saracci, Richard. 2007. "Epidemiological Concepts Pre-1950 and Their Relation to Work in the Second Half of the Century." In *The Development of Modern Epidemiology: Personal Reports from Those Who Were There*, edited by W. W. Holland, J. Olsen, and C. du V. Florey, 31–38. Oxford: Oxford University Press.

Scheper-Hughes, Nancy. 1984. "Infant Mortality and Infant Care: Cultural and Economic Constraints on Nurturing in Northeast Brazil." *Social Science & Medicine* 19 (5): 535–546.

———. 1995. "The Primacy of the Ethical: Propositions for a Militant Anthropology." *Current Anthropology* 36 (3): 409–440.

Scott, James. 1998. *Seeing Like a State: How Certain Schemes to Improve the Human Condition Have Failed*. New Haven, CT: Yale University Press.

Scott-Smith, Tom. 2013. "The Fetishism of Humanitarian Objects and the Management of Malnutrition in Emergencies." *Third World Quarterly* 34 (5): 913–928. https://doi.org/http://dx.doi.org/10.1080/01436597.2013.800749.

Scrimshaw, Nevin S., Carl E. Taylor, and John E. Gordon. 1959. "Interactions of Nutrition and Infection." *American Journal of the Medical Sciences* 237 (3): 367–403.

———, eds. 1968. *Interactions of Nutrition and Infection*. Geneva: World Health Organization.

Seekings, Jeremy, and Nicoli Nattrass. 2002. "Class, Distribution and Redistribution in Post-Apartheid South Africa." *Transformation: Critical Perspectives on Southern Africa* 50 (1): 1–30. https://doi.org/10.1353/trn.2003.0014.

———. 2005. *Class, Race and Inequality in South Africa.* New Haven, CT: Yale University Press.

Shisana, Olive, Demetre Labadarios, Thomas Rehle, Leickness Simbayi, Khangelani Zuma, Ali Dhansay, Priscilla Reddy, et al. 2013. *South African National Health and Nutrition Examination Survey (SANHANES-1).* Cape Town: HSRC Press.

Shostak, Sara, and Margot Moinester. 2015. "The Missing Piece of the Puzzle? Measuring the Environment in the Postgenomic Moment." In *Postgenomics: Perspectives on Biology and the Genome,* edited by S. Richardson and H. Stevens, 192–209. Durham, NC: Duke University Press.

Signorello, Lisa B., and Dimitrios Trichopoulos. 1998. "Perinatal Determinants of Adult Cardiovascular Disease and Cancer." *Scandinavian Journal of Social Medicine* 26: 161–165.

Simone, AbdouMaliq. 2004. "People as Infrastructure: Intersecting Fragments in Johannesburg." *Public Culture* 16 (3): 407–429.

Singer, Merrill. 1995. "Beyond the Ivory Tower: Critical Praxis in Medical Anthropology." *Medical Anthropology Quarterly* 9 (1): 80–106.

Singer, Merrill, Nicola Bulled, Bayla Ostrach, and Emily Mendenhall. 2017. "Syndemics and the Biosocial Conception of Health." *The Lancet* 389 (10072): 941–950.

Skeen, S., M. Tomlinson, C. L. Ward, L. Cluver, and J. M. Lachman. 2015. "Early Intervention: A Foundation for Lifelong Violence Prevention." *South African Crime Quarterly* 51: 05–07. https://doi.org/10.4314/sacq.v51i1.1.

Skuse, Andrew, and Thomas Cousins. 2007. "Spaces of Resistance: Informal Settlement, Communication and Community Organisation in a Cape Town Township." *Urban Studies* 44 (5): 979–995. https://doi.org/10.1080/00420980701256021.

Smit, Warren, Ariane de Lannoy, Robert V. H. Dover, Estelle V. Lambert, Naomi Levitt, and Vanessa Watson. 2015. "Making Unhealthy Places: The Built Environment and Non-Communicable Diseases in Khayelitsha, Cape Town." *Health & Place* 35: 11–18. https://doi.org/10.1016/j.healthplace.2015.06.006.

Smith, David F., ed. 1997. *Nutrition in Britain: Science, Scientists and Politics in the Twentieth Century.* London: Routledge.

Social Justice Coalition and Ndifuna Ukwazi. 2014. *Our Toilets Are Dirty: Report of The Social Audit into the Janitorial Service for Communal Flush Toilets in Khayelitsha, Cape Town.* Cape Town: Social Justice Coalition and Ndifuna Ukwazi.

Solomon, Harris. 2016. *Metabolic Living: Food, Fat, and the Absorption of Illness in India.* Durham, NC: Duke University Press.

South African Vitamin A Consultative Group. 1995. *Children Aged 6–71 Months in South Africa, 1994: Their Anthropometric, Vitamin A, Iron and Immunisation Coverage Status.* Johannesburg: SAVACG.

Spiegel, Andrew, and Anthony Mehlwana. 1997. *Family as Social Network: Kinship and Sporadic Migrancy in the Western Cape's Khayelitsha.* Pretoria: Human Sciences Research Council.

Spiegel, Andrew, Vanessa Watson, and Peter Wilkinson. 1996. "Domestic Diversity and Fluidity among Some African Households in Greater Cape Town." *Social Dynamics* 22 (1): 7–30. https://doi.org/10.1080/02533959608458599.

Sridhar, Devi. 2008. *The Battle against Hunger: Choice, Circumstance, and the World Bank.* Oxford: Oxford University Press.

Stadler, Jonathan J., Sinead Delany, and Mdu Mntambo. 2008. "Women's Perceptions and Experiences of HIV Prevention Trials in Soweto, South Africa." *Social Science and Medicine* 66 (1): 189–200. https://doi.org/10.1016/j.socscimed.2007.08.021.

Stadler, Jonathan J., Fiona Scorgie, Ariane van der Straten, and Eirik Saethre. 2015. "Adherence and the Lie in a HIV Prevention Clinical Trial." *Medical Anthropology* 35 (6): 503–516.

Statistics South Africa. 2008. "Measuring Poverty in South Africa: Methodological Report on the Development of the Poverty Lines for Statistical Reporting." Accessed February 11, 2014. https://www.justice.gov.za/commissions/feeshet/hearings/set5/set05-d1-DrPaliLehohla -MeasuringPovertyReport.pdf.

———. 2013. "City of Cape Town—2011 Census—Khayelitsha Health District." Accessed February 11, 2014. https://resource.capetown.gov.za/documentcentre/Documents/Maps %20and%20statistics/Khayelitsha%20Health%20District.pdf.

Stellmach, Darryl. 2016. "Coordination in Crisis: The Practice of Medical Humanitarian Emergency." PhD diss., University of Oxford.

Stephenson, Judith, Nicola Heslehurst, Jennifer Hall, Danielle A. J. M. Schoenaker, Jayne Hutchinson, Janet E. Cade, Lucilla Poston, et al. 2018. "Before the Beginning: Nutrition and Lifestyle in the Preconception Period and Its Importance for Future Health." *The Lancet* 391 (10132): 1830–1841. https://doi.org/10.1016/S0140-6736(18)30311-8.

Stevens, Hallam, and Sarah S. Richardson. "Beyond the Genome." In *Postgenomics: Perspectives on Biology and the Genome*, edited by S. S. Richardson and H. Stevens, 210–231. Durham, NC: Duke University Press.

Steyn, Krisela, Jean Fourie, and Norman Temple, eds. 2006. *Chronic Diseases of Lifestyle in South Africa: 1995–2005*. Cape Town: South African Medical Research Council.

Steyn, Melissa. 2001. *Whiteness Just Isn't What It Used to Be: White Identity in a Changing South Africa*. Albany: State University of New York Press.

Steyn, Nelia P., Johanna H. Nel, W. Parker, Rosemary Ayah, and Dorcus Mbithe. 2012. "Urbanisation and the Nutrition Transition: A Comparison of Diet and Weight Status of South African and Kenyan Women." *Scandinavian Journal of Public Health* 40 (3): 229–238.

Storey, Angela. 2014. "Making Experience Legible: Spaces of Participation and the Construction of Knowledge in Khayelitsha." *Politikon* 41 (3): 403–420.

Street, Alice. 2012. "Affective Infrastructure: Hospital Landscapes of Hope and Failure." *Space and Culture* 15 (1): 44–56.

———. 2014. *Biomedicine in an Unstable Place: Infrastructure and Personhood in a Papua New Guinean Hospital*. Durham, NC: Duke University Press.

Summers, Carol. 1991. "Intimate Colonialism: The Imperial Production of Reproduction in Uganda, 1907–1925." *Signs* 16 (4): 787–807.

Surplus People's Project (Cape Town, South Africa). 1984. *Khayelitsha: New Home—Old Story: A Dossier of Forced Removals of Cape Town's African Population*. Cape Town: Surplus People's Project.

Susser, Ida. 2010. "The Anthropologist as Social Critic." *Current Anthropology* 51 (S2): S227–S233. https://doi.org/10.1086/653127.

Susser, Mervyn. 1985. "Epidemiology in the United States after World War II: The Evolution of Technique." *Epidemiologic Reviews* 7: 147–177.

Suzman, Susan M. 1994. "Names as Pointers: Zulu Personal Naming Practices." *Language in Society* 23 (2): 253–272. https://doi.org/10.1017/S0047404500017851.

Szyf, Moshe. 2015. "'Nongenetic' Inheritance and Transgenerational Epigenetics." *Trends in Molecular Medicine* 21 (2): 134–144.

Talbot, Kirsten, and Michael Quayle. 2010. "The Perils of Being a Nice Guy: Contextual Variation in Five Young Women's Constructions of Acceptable Hegemonic and Alternative Masculinities." *Men and Masculinities* 13 (2): 255–278. https://doi.org/10.1177/1097184X09350408.

Taussig, Karen Sue, Klaus Hoeyer, and Stefan Helmreich. 2013. "The Anthropology of Potentiality in Biomedicine." *Current Anthropology* 54 (S7): S3–S14. https://doi.org/10.1086/671401.

Temple, Norman J., and Nelia P. Steyn. 2009. "Food Prices and Energy Density as Barriers to Healthy Food Choices in Cape Town." *Journal of Hunger and Environmental Nutrition* 4: 203–213.

Thayer, Zaneta M., and Christopher W. Kuzawa. 2011. "Biological Memories of Past Environments: Epigenetic Pathways to Health Disparities." *Epigenetics* 6 (7): 798–803. https://doi.org/10.4161/epi.6.7.16222.

Theidon, Kimberley. 2015. "Hidden in Plain Sight: Children Born of Wartime Sexual Violence." *Current Anthropology* 56 (S12): S191–S200.

Thompson, Warren S. 1929. "Danger Spots in World Population." *American Journal of Sociology*, 34: 959–975.

Thornton, Robert J., and Mamphele Ramphele. 1989. "Community: Concept and Practice in South Africa." *Critique of Anthropology* 9 (1): 75–87. https://doi.org/10.1177/0308275X8900900106.

Thurow, Roger. 2016. *The First 1000 Days: A Crucial Time for Mothers and Children—and the World*. New York: Perseus Books.

Ticktin, Miriam. 2011. *Casualties of Care: Immigration and the Politics of Humanitarianism in France*. Berkeley: University of California Press.

Tilley, Helen. 2011. *Africa as a Living Laboratory: Empire, Development, and the Problem of Scientific Knowledge, 1870–1950*. London: University of Chicago Press.

Timmermans, Stefan, and Rene Almeling. 2009. "Objectification, Standardization, and Commodification in Health Care: A Conceptual Readjustment." *Social Science & Medicine* 69 (1): 21–27. https://doi.org/10.1016/j.socscimed.2009.04.020.

Timmermans, Stefan, and Marc Berg. 1997. "Standardization in Action: Achieving Local Universality through Medical Protocols." *Social Studies of Science* 27 (2): 273–305.

Tobi, Elmar W., L. H. Lumey, Rudolf P. Talens, Dennis Kremer, Hein Putter, Aryeh D. Stein, P. Eline Slagboom, et al. 2009. "DNA Methylation Differences after Exposure to Prenatal Famine Are Common and Timing- and Sex-Specific." *Human Molecular Genetics* 18 (21): 4046–4053. https://doi.org/10.1093/hmg/ddp353.

Tolwinski, Kasia. 2019. "Fraught Claims at the Intersection of Biology and Sociality: Managing Controversy in the Neuroscience of Poverty and Adversity." *Social Studies of Science* 49 (2): 141–161. https://doi.org/10.1177/0306312719839149.

Tomlinson, Mark. 2012. "'Toxic Poverty'—Improving Maternal, Infant and Child Health in Contexts of High Adversity." Inaugural lecture, University of Stellenbosch, November.

Tuck, Eve. 2009. "Suspending Damage: A Letter to Communities." *Harvard Educational Review* 79: 409–427.

Ulijaszek, Stanley J. 1996. "Long-Term Consequences of Early Environments on Human Growth: A Developmental Perspective." In *Long-Term Consequences of Early Environment: Growth, Development and the Lifespan Developmental Perspective*, edited by C. J. K. Henry and Stanley J. Ulijaszek, 2–3. Cambridge: Cambridge University Press.

Ulijaszek, Stanley J., Sarah Elton, and Neil Mann. 2012. *Evolving Human Nutrition: Implications for Public Health*. Cambridge: Cambridge University Press.

United Nations. 2000. "United Nations Millennium Declaration." Accessed 18 July, 2023. https://www.un.org/en/development/desa/population/migration/generalassembly/docs/globalcompact/A_RES_55_2.pdf.

Valdez, Natali. 2021. *Weighing the Future: Race, Science and Pregnancy Trials in the Postgenomic Era*. Oakland: University of California Press.

Valdez, Natali, and Daisy Deomampo. 2019. "Centering Race and Racism in Reproduction." *Medical Anthropology* 38 (7): 551–559.

Van der Merwe, M. T., Nigel Crowther, Glen P. Schlaphoff, I. P. Gray, B. I. Joffe, and P. N. Lonroth. 2000. "Evidence for Insulin Resistance in Black Women from South Africa." *International Journal of Obesity and Related Metabolic Disorders* 24: 1340–1346.

Van der Merwe, M. T., and M. S. Pepper. 2006. "Obesity in South Africa." *Obesity Reviews* 7 (4): 315–322.

Van Esterik, Penny. 2002. "Contemporary Trends in Infant Feeding Research." *Annual Review of Anthropology* 31 (2002): 257–278. https://doi.org/10.1146/annurev.anthro.31.040402.085428.

———. 2013. "The Politics of Breastfeeding: An Advocacy Update." In *Food and Culture: A Reader*, 3rd ed., edited by Carole Counihan and Penny van Esterik, 51–30. London: Routledge.

Van Hollen, Cecilia. 2011. "Breast or Bottle? HIV-Positive Women's Responses to Global Health Policy on Infant Feeding in India." *Medical Anthropology Quarterly* 25 (4): 499–518.

Van Wyk, Ilana. 2014. *The Universal Church of the Kingdom of God in South Africa: A Church of Strangers*. Cambridge: Cambridge University Press.

Vaughan, Megan. 1988. "Measuring Crisis in Maternal and Child Health: An Historical Perspective." In *Women's Health and Apartheid: The Health of Women and Children and the Future of Progressive Primary Health Care in Southern Africa: Proceedings of the Third Workshop of the Project on Poverty, Health, and the State in Southern Africa*, edited by Marcia Wright, Zena Stein, and Jean Scandlyn, 130–142. New York: Columbia University.

———. 1991. *Curing Their Ills: Colonial Power and African Illness*. Stanford, CA: Stanford University Press.

Verissimo, Jumoke. 2019. "On the Politics of Italics." Literary Hub. https://lithub.com/on-the-politics-of-italics.

Victora, Cesar G., Linda Adair, Caroline Fall, Pedro C. Hallal, Reynaldo Martorell, Linda Richter, and Harshpal Singh Sachdev. 2008. "Maternal and Child Undernutrition: Consequences for Adult Health and Human Capital." *Lancet* 371 (9609): 340–357. https://doi.org/10.1016/S0140-6736(07)61692-4.

Vlok, Marie E. 1991. *Manual of Community Nursing and Communicable Diseases: A Textbook for South African Students*. Lansdowne: Juta.

Von Schnitzler, Antina. 2013. "Traveling Technologies: Infrastructure, Ethical Regimes, and the Materiality of Politics in South Africa." *Cultural Anthropology* 28(4): 670–693.

Vorster, Hester H., Lesley T. Bourne, Christina S. Venter, and Welma Oosthuizen. 1999. "Contribution of Nutrition to the Health Transition in Developing Countries: A Framework for Research and Intervention." *Nutrition Reviews* 57 (11): 341–349.

Vorster, Hester H., Annamarie Kruger, and Barrie M. Margetts. 2011. "The Nutrition Transition in Africa: Can It Be Steered into a More Positive Direction?" *Nutrients* 3 (4): 429–441.

Waddington, Conrad H. 1942. "The Epigenotype." *Endeavour* 41 (1): 18–20.

———. 1968. "The Basic Ideas of Biology." In *Towards a Theoretical Biology*, vol. 1, *Prolegomena*, 1–32. Edinburgh: Edinburgh University Press.

Wadsworth, Mike E., Harrison A. Cripps, R. E. Midwinter, and J. R. Colley. 1985. "Blood Pressure in a National Birth Cohort at the Age of 36 Related to Social and Familial Factors, Smoking, and Body Mass." *British Medical Journal* 291 (6508): 1534–1538.

Walker, A. R., F. Adam, and B. F. Walker. 2001. "World Pandemic of Obesity: The Situation in Southern African Populations." *Public Health* 115 (6): 368–372.

Walker, A. R. P., B. F. Walker, A. J. Walker, and H. H. Vorster. 1989. "Low Frequency of Adverse Sequelae of Obesity in South African Rural Black Women." *International Journal for Vitamin and Nutrition Research* 59 (2): 224–228.

Ward, Catherine L., Christopher Mikton, Lucie Cluver, Peter Cooper, Frances Gardner, Judy Hutchings, Jamie McLaren Lachmann, et al. 2014. "Parenting for Lifelong Health: From South Africa to Other Low- and Middle-Income Countries." *Early Childhood Matters* 122: 49–53.

Warin, Megan, Jaya Keaney, Emma Kowal, and Henrietta Byrne. 2022. "Circuits of Time: Enacting Postgenomics in Indigenous Australia." *Body & Society* 29 (2): 20–48. https://doi.org/10.1177/1357034X211070041.

Warin, Megan, Vivienne Moore, Michael Davies, and Stanley J. Ulijaszek. 2015. "Epigenetics and Obesity: The Reproduction of Habitus through Intracellular and Social Environments." *Body & Society* 22 (4): 53–78.

Warin, Megan, Tanya Zivkovic, Vivienne Moore, and Michael Davies. 2012. "Mothers as Smoking Guns: Fetal Overnutrition and the Reproduction of Obesity." *Feminism & Psychology* 22 (3): 360–375. https://doi.org/10.1177/0959353512445359.

Waterland, Robert A., and Cutberto Garza. 1999. "Potential Mechanisms of Metabolic Imprinting that Lead to Chronic Disease." *American Journal of Clinical Nutrition* 69 (2): 179–197.

Waterland, Robert A., and Karin B. Michels. 2007. "Epigenetic Epidemiology of the Developmental Origins Hypothesis." *Annual Review of Nutrition* 27: 363–388. https://doi.org/10.1146/annurev.nutr.27.061406.093705.

Watson, James D., and Francis H. C. Crick. 1953. "Genetical Implications of the Structure of Deoxyribonucleic Acid." *Nature* 171: 964–967.

Wendland, Claire L. 2010. *A Heart for the Work: Journeys through an African Medical School.* Chicago: Chicago University Press.

———. 2019. "Physician Anthropologists." *Annual Review of Anthropology* 48 (1): 18–85. https://doi.org/10.1146/annurev-anthro-102218-011338.

Western Cape Government Health. 2014. *Healthcare 2030: The Road to Wellness.* [Cape Town: Western Cape Department of Health]. https://www.westerncape.gov.za/assets/departments/health/healthcare2030_0.pdf.

Western Cape Government. 2016. First 1000 Days Campaign. Accessed January 20, 2017. https://www.westerncape.gov.za/general-publication/first-1-000-days-campaign.

Wheeler, Erica. 1985. "To Feed or to Educate: Labelling in Targeted Nutrition Interventions." In *Labelling in Development Policy*, edited by Geoff Wood, 475–483. London: Sage Publications.

White, Hylton. 2001. "Tempora et Mores: Family Values and the Possessions of a Post-Apartheid Countryside." *Journal of Religion in Africa* 31(4): 45–79.

Wild, Christopher Paul. 2005. "Complementing the Genome with an 'Exposome': The Outstanding Challenge of Environmental Exposure Measurement in Molecular Epidemiology." *Cancer Epidemiology, Biomarkers & Prevention* 14 (8): 1847–1850.

Williams, Paul, and Ian Taylor. 2010. "Neoliberalism and the Political Economy of the 'New' South Africa." *New Political Economy* 5 (1): 21–40.

World Bank. 2006. *Repositioning Nutrition as Central to Development: A Strategy for Large-Scale Action.* Washington DC: World Bank Publications. https://documents1.worldbank.org/curated/en/185651468175733998/pdf/574890WP0Nutri1iewofororeport034775.pdf.

———. 2019. "Gini Index—South Africa." World Bank Data. October 6, 2019. https://data.worldbank.org/indicator/SI.POV.GINI?locations=ZA.

World Health Organization. 2007. *HIV and Infant Feeding: Update Based on the Technical Consultation Held on Behalf of the Inter-Agency Team (IATT) on Prevention of HIV Infections in Pregnant Women, Mothers and Their Infants, Geneva, 2–7 October 2006.* Geneva: World Health Organization.

———. 2018. *Noncommunicable Diseases Country Profiles 2018.* Geneva: World Health Organization. 2018. https://apps.who.int/iris/handle/10665/274512.

World Obesity Federation. 2019. *Atlas of Childhood Obesity.* London: World Obesity Federation.

Wylie, Diana. 2001. *Starving on a Full Stomach: Hunger and the Triumph of Cultural Racism in South Africa.* Charlottesville: University of Virginia Press.

Yates-Doerr, Emily. 2011. "Bodily Betrayal: Love and Anger in the Time of Epigenetics." In *A Companion to the Anthropology of the Body and Embodiment*, edited by Frances E. Mascia-Lees, 292–306. Chichester: Wiley-Blackwell.

———. 2015a. *The Weight of Obesity: Hunger and Global Health in Postwar Guatemala.* Berkeley: University of California Press.

———. 2015b. "Intervals of Confidence: Uncertain Accounts of Global Hunger." *BioSocieties* 10 (2): 229–246.

Yehuda, Rachel, and Amy Lehrner. 2018. "Intergenerational Transmission of Trauma Effects: Putative Role of Epigenetic Mechanisms." *World Psychiatry* 17: 243–257.

Zarowsky, Christina, Slim Haddad, and Vinh-Kim Nguyen. 2013. "Beyond 'Vulnerable Groups': Contexts and Dynamics of Vulnerability." *Global Health Promotion* 20 (3): 3–9. https://doi.org/10.1177/1757975912470062.

Ziegler, John B., Richard O. Johnson, David A. Cooper, and Julian Gold. 1985. "Postnatal Transmission of Aids-Associated Retrovirus from Mother to Infant." *The Lancet* 325 (8434): 896–898. https://doi.org/10.1016/S0140-6736(85)91673-3.

Zola, Irving. 1972. "Medicine as an Institution of Social Control." *Sociological Review* 20: 487–504.

INDEX

Page numbers in italics refer to figures or tables; page numbers followed by "n" refer to endnotes.

ABOUT THE AUTHOR

MICHELLE PENTECOST is a South African physician-anthropologist. She completed her medical training at the University of Cape Town and her doctorate in anthropology at the University of Oxford. Pentecost has a decade of work experience as a clinician in South Africa. Her research and publication record reflects her interest in the interdisciplinary domains of clinical medicine, anthropology, science and technology studies, and the medical humanities. Her work has been funded by UK Research and Innovation, the British Academy, and the Wellcome Trust.